HOMOEOPATHY:
HEART & SOUL

Dr. KEITH M. SOUTER
MB, ChB, MRCGP, MHMA

Homoeopathy: Heart & Soul

Treatment for Emotional Problems

Index compiled by Lyn Greenwood

MOTILAL BANARSIDASS PUBLISHERS
PRIVATE LIMITED • DELHI

First Indian Edition: Delhi, 1996

First published in Great Britain in 1993 by The C.W. Daniel Company Limited, 1 Church Path, Saffron Walden, Essex, CB10 1JP, England

ISBN: 81-208-1415-0 (Cloth)
ISBN: 81-208-1419-3 (Paper)

For Rachel, Kate, Ruth and Andrew, who put up with me as I explored the emotional jungle for 'Heart and Soul'

Also available at:

MOTILAL BANARSIDASS
41 U.A. Bungalow Road, Jawahar Nagar, Delhi 110 007
120 Royapettah High Road, Mylapore, Madras 600 004
16 St. Mark's Road, Bangalore 560 001
8 Camac Street, Calcutta 700 017
Ashok Rajpath, Patna 800 004
Chowk, Varanasi 221 001

PRINTED IN INDIA
BY JAINENDRA PRAKASH JAIN AT SHRI JAINENDRA PRESS, A-45 NARAINA, PHASE I, NEW DELHI 110 028
AND PUBLISHED BY NARENDRA PRAKASH JAIN FOR MOTILAL BANARSIDASS PUBLISHERS PRIVATE LIMITED, BUNGALOW ROAD, DELHI 110 007

Contents

Introduction

Emotional problems are part and parcel of life. However, while some people seem able to ride any emotional storm, others never seem to reach a state of calm, but carry a burden of storm damage within their psyche.

Anxiety, depression, phobias, insomnia – these are just some of the problems which face people in this more and more complicated world in which we live. Indeed, it is estimated that psychological and emotional problems account for up to 20 per cent of all *primary* diagnoses in General Practice. When psychological testing of *all patients* is performed, however, a marked psychological or emotional component is found in at least 70 per cent of illness.

Most practitioners suspect that these figures, amazing though they seem, still only represent the tip of the iceberg. Many people never seek help from any sort of health adviser. These 'brave soldiers' battle on valiantly (or so they perceive), when in actual fact they probably end up living around their emotional problem.

The good news is that there is much that can be done for emotional problems with homoeopathy. Since this gentle form of treatment is very individual, and works by matching up the remedy to the pattern of emotional problem, it is ideal for calming the troubled waters of the mind. It does not, of course, solve the problems which cause the emotional problem, but it balances one so that things can be put into perspective, so that the problem can be rationally solved.

This book is not intended to replace orthodox medical advice or treatment. Where it is essential to seek medical advice then this is mentioned throughout the text. Above all, it is important not to stop taking any prescribed medication without medical advice.

There are three parts to this book. Part One covers the range of emotional problems, their importance in homoeopathy, and the principles of the homoeopathic method. Part Two deals with specific emotional problems. Finally, Part Three consists of a Materia Medica, an outline of all the profiles of the remedies mentioned in the book. This is followed by a Therapeutic Index, an A–Z of common emotions and emotional problems detailing the remedies which work well with them.

Flow charts are also included in order to help differentiate remedies quickly in most of the treatment groups. These are very straightforward and, while not being in any way definitive, may be of help for rapid reference.

To get the best out of this book it is as well to read through Part One to understand the basic principles. The appropriate chapter in Part Two will then guide one to the best, or most frequently indicated remedies for that problem. The Materia Medica then gives a fuller analysis of the particular remedies. Finally, as a quick reference tool, the Therapeutic Index will indicate the likeliest remedies in most emotional problems. Again, the Materia Medica allows the final check to be made.

Our emotions govern our lives. As we shall see, they affect the way we think and the way we feel. Homoeopathy, by aiming directly at those emotions, reharmonises and rebalances the individual. It is the gentle persuader – a subtle form of treatment which acts at the very heart and soul of the problem.

Keith Souter

PART ONE

EMOTIONS *and* HOMOEOPATHY

CHAPTER 1

Our Emotional Life

Some feelings are to mortals given,
With less of earth in them than heaven.
Sir Walter Scott, *The Lady of the Lake*.

There are two things which are common to all human beings. Thought and emotions.

The two things are often intimately related, because our emotions may affect the way we think, just as the content of our thoughts can make us feel emotional.

Essentially, an emotion is the experience of a feeling or mood, as a result of which we may be driven to act or think in a particular manner. In addition, we may experience physical sensations which then become associated with that emotion.

Usually, there is an obvious trigger for the emotion, some rational explanation as to why we feel as we do. For example, upon the anniversary of the death of her husband a young widow sinks into a bout of depression and starts to weep. Similarly, a schoolboy faced with reading an essay in front of the whole school may well feel frightened and experience a quickening of the heart and a tendency to perspire. Most people could empathise with these two examples.

Why we experience these emotions at all is hard to explain. It is not as if they are learned in the same way that we learn facts and skills. The experience of anger is probably the same for a toddler living in the flatlands of Holland as it is for an old man who has lived his life in the foothills of the Himalayas. The intensity of the emotion, the expression of it and the cause may all be different, yet if they were able to compare their 'feelings,' it is likely that they would be talking about the same thing.

Undoubtedly some emotions serve a useful purpose, in that they may help us to focus our minds in a particular manner. Others may be useful in that they make us act in an appropriate way. In this, they could be compared to other feelings like pain, which make us act in a manner to reduce the pain, or remove the cause.

Unfortunately, when an emotion persists for longer than one would expect from the original triggering stimulus, then the conditions are ripe for developing an '*emotional problem.*'

And like pain which persists after the painful trigger has gone or has healed, the emotional problem can produce all sorts of secondary effects which ruin one's sense of well-being.

Feelings, sensations and actions – the components of emotion

Scientists have had a difficult time defining what an emotion is. In general, however, they consider it from the following three aspects – psychology, physiology and behaviour.

Let us pick the emotion of fear, for example. The individual finding himself in some dangerous situation is likely to have the 'feeling' that something unpleasant is about to happen. He may notice that he begins to perspire, his heart races and he feels butterflies in the stomach. All of this may cause him to want to escape from the situation, which he may well do by running away. Alternatively, he may feel that he must overcome the fearful situation, so he prepares to fight.

The psychological component of this emotion is the feeling of impending unpleasantness. Physiologically, the adrenal glands pump out adrenaline, the hormone which causes a speeding up of the heart, an increase in perspiration, a drying up of the mouth and an alteration in the motility of the bowels. Essentially, the physiological effect is to prepare the body for 'fight or flight.' And so finally, the way the individual acts or behaves, marks the behavioural component.

When you consider emotions in this way it seems likely that the sequence begins with the triggering stimulus producing the psychological '*feeling*,' which then produces the physical '*sensation*,' resulting in the characteristic *action* or *behaviour* one associates with the particular emotion. Thus, we feel sad, then cry; or we feel happy, then laugh. Not all psychologists would agree, however.

According to the *James-Lange Law*, first formulated in 1884 by the American psychologist William James and the Norwegian physiologist Lange, the bodily sensations come first. As a result, they trigger off the psychological feeling which makes us experience the emotion.

When one considers the so-called major emotions, then this seems plausible. Going back to the original example of fear, the bodily release of adrenaline could easily trigger the 'fight or flight' reaction, thereby producing the feeling of 'fear.' On the other hand, it seems naïve to imagine that a stimulus makes one cry, and that because of the crying you feel sad.

But if you follow it all through you can soon get tied down in chicken and egg arguments. The important thing to appreciate is that the emotions mark an obvious point at which mind and body functions become one. Later, we will see that this is precisely why homoeopathy is so appropriate for dealing with problems of the emotions.

The range of emotions

Man has always recognised the differing emotions to which he has been subject. The religious beliefs of the Ancients affirms this, since the names of many of their deities have passed down to us. For example, the Greeks believed that Ares, the god of war, was always accompanied by his son *Phobos* (Fright), and that the god *Pan* delighted in inflicting sudden terror attacks upon lonely travellers. Herein we can see two common emotional problems – *phobias* and *panic attacks*.

To the Ancient Chinese the emotions were considered an integral part of life. According to Traditional Chinese Medicine, however, if one of *the seven emotions* persists over a long time, illness will result. Within the system the relevant emotions are considered to be – happiness, anger, worry, pensiveness, sadness, fear and terror. Interestingly, it is believed that it is not only the negative emotions which can cause problems. Being happy for too long, or thinking too hard for too long can also produce illness.

Although the Chinese seven emotions, plus their concept of 'frustration,' seem to cover a lot of ground, we in the West seem to be afflicted with the additional negative emotions of guilt, jealousy and hatred. And of course, people all over the world are affected by love, either returned or unrequited.

The range of emotional problems

Anxiety and depression are the two commonest emotional problems faced by people in the West, together accounting for about sixty per cent of emotional problems. The causes vary from person to person, as does the degree of the emotion. Anxiety ranges from the slightly nervous anticipation of an event to the crippling panic attack. Similarly, depression varies from the slightly down in the dumps feeling to the depths of despair. Self-destructive actions, possibly even suicidal attempts may accompany the latter.

IT IS IMPORTANT THAT IF SOMEONE FEELS LIKE HARMING THEMSELVES, OR OF ENDING THEIR LIVES – THEY SHOULD CONSULT A DOCTOR IMMEDIATELY.

Phobias affect about 15 to 20 per cent of the population. Essentially, they are states in which an excessive amount of fear is felt when one comes in contact with an object or situation which in itself does not really pose any danger. Despite the fact that the sufferer knows this, they are unable to face the situation, so they avoid it. Thus people who fear crowds (*agoraphobia*) may never leave their homes; those who hate enclosed spaces (*claustrophobia*) may never be able to travel in a lift, and those with very specific fears – eg, of cats – may never be able to visit a house without first ascertaining that there is no kitten in the vicinity. Truly, it can be an incredibly limiting problem.

Anger is something which virtually everyone experiences from time to time. For some people, however, it can come on so suddenly that they find themselves ostracized. Life for them can be a continual strain as they struggle to control their temper. Relationships, jobs, even simple social engagements can fall foul of the sudden rages.

To a lesser degree, irritability can produce strain upon the individual. It can flare up at the most trivial of causes, or it can become so chronic that the whole outlook upon life becomes cynical.

The green-eyed monster of jealousy can rear its ugly head at any stage of life, from infancy to old age. Sometimes it bobs back under the surface after a quick sortie, but sometimes its malevolent gaze bores into the unfortunate to take over their life.

Guilt is one of the most destructive of emotions. Indeed, according to psychoanalytic theory it is one of the main factors involved in the development of illness. In order to avoid the emotion of guilt, the mind is thought to operate a number of unconscious mental defence mechanisms which allow the individual to cope with feelings which would normally make him feel guilty. We shall return to this topic in Chapter 5.

There are of course times in life when one is at a low ebb. For women the premenstrual phase is a recurring time when there is the potential to go out of balance. Between ovulation and the onset of the menstrual flow there are profound hormonal changes taking place. In addition, dietary intake may vary from the usual to cause mineral and electrolyte fluctuations. At this vulnerable time many women suffer from the premenstrual syndrome (PMS). For a proportion it is a time to be dreaded, because many different and uncharacteristic emotions may be experienced, ranging from depression to jealousy and violent tantrums.

The image one has of the body is very important. If the image is poor, then self esteem is also likely to be poor. Sometimes that image becomes distorted, leading to the eating disorders of *anorexia nervosa* and *bulimia*. They are not problems to be minimised.

IF SOMEONE'S THOUGHTS SEEM TO BE DOMINATED BY SLIMMING, DIETING OR, CONVERSELY BY THE DESIRE TO BINGE EAT, THEN A MEDICAL OPINION SHOULD BE SOUGHT.

When the mind is beset with cares and worries it is common to find sleep difficult. To 'normal sleepers' the plight of the insomniac is incomprehensible. Unfortunately, many sufferers end up having their problem being compounded when they start taking sleeping tablets. Sadly, as many people know to their cost, it does not take many such tablets to create a drug dependency problem.

And indeed, the 'social habits' which people take up to help them 'relax', are coping mechanisms which so often prove to be double-edged. They become addictions which the individual feels are necessary to their life. Smoking, alcohol, caffeine, benzodiazepines – all of them may initially seem to help the individual, yet it is at a price.

And finally, there is love. The emotion which they say makes the world go round. It has many forms, many expressions, many consequences. It can be sweet or bittersweet. For some it can truly become a love-sickness.

Just as the emotions are many and diverse, so can the number of emotional problems be legion. Fortunately, while the source of the problem may seem to be insoluble, the state of mind is not. It is possible to restore balance and harmony so that one can look at the problem calmly – and hopefully deal with it properly.

Vulnerable constitutions

Everyone knows of people who could be described as:- 'bad-tempered,' 'a born worrier,' 'a life-long depressive,' 'a guilt-carrier,' 'a moaner,' etc, etc. In other words while some people may seem to ride any emotional storm, or only pass transiently though an emotion, others will react in a way typical to them.

You do not have to be a psychiatrist, a psychologist or an expert observer of human nature to appreciate that some people seem to be more vulnerable than others. Faced with a stressful situation, be it environmental, physical or emotional, they are liable to respond true to their past form. Thus, using the examples above, if five people representative of those groups met with the same trauma, they might respectively react with:- anger, anxiety, sadness, self-reproach, self-pity.

It seems that people react according to their constitutional types. Being able to pin this down is obviously of immense importance, since if one can predict the way someone is liable to react, then the pattern of their emotional response will suggest the best way of dealing with it.

As we shall see later there are often other indicators which alert one to particular response patterns. It may be that someone reacts to weather in a particular manner, prefers certain foods, tends to get particular ailments, or even have certain physical features.

Of course, someone who tends to feel depressed a lot of the time can also respond to events or situations with anger, anxiety, or self-reproach. One emotion may naturally lead to another, or it may be the 'appropriate' emotion at the time. Sometimes these mixed emotions can be very troublesome, but like the Gordion knot it is possible to unravel and deal with them appropriately.

Homoeopathy, a holistic approach

As I mentioned at the beginning of the chapter emotions have several components. The emotional feeling is often accompanied by the physical sensation and a behavioural pattern. This means that the emotion has effects on the mind, body and environment. This being the case it should be clear that the best way of approaching the problem is to study the feeling, the sensation and the behavioural pattern as parts of one picture. Essentially this is the holistic approach.

As we shall see in the next three chapters since this is the very basis of homoeopathy, it is one of the most logical ways of coping with emotional problems.

CHAPTER 2

The Principles of Homoeopathy

Similia similibus curentur
(Let like be treated by like)

Homoeopathy is a gentle form of Medicine which was known to the Ancient Greeks, a fact mirrored by its derivation from the Greek *homoios*, meaning 'like,' and *pathos*, meaning 'suffering.' Essentially it means treating like with like.

The great physician Hippocrates first taught that there were two ways of treating a patient. Either one could cure by 'contraries,' or by 'similarities.' That is, one could either give medication to counteract symptoms – *the law of contraries*; or medication which had the ability to produce the same symptoms as those suffered by the ill person – *the law of similars*.

In both cases he believed that the physician was merely creating the right conditions for the inner healing power, *Vis Medicatrix Naturae* to bring about the cure.

Over the centuries physicians continued to practice both types of Medicine, although it was not until the 18th Century that the similars principle became formulated into a distinct system of Medicine. The founder of this school of thought was an eccentric genius by the name of Samuel Hahnemann.

Dr Samuel Hahnemann

The son of a china-painter in the famous Meissen pottery works, Samuel Christian Hahnemann (1755–1843) qualified as a doctor from the University of Erlangen in 1779. After several unhappy years in practice, he became thoroughly disenchanted with the rather brutal and dubious medical treatments of the day. In a manner which was typical of his nature he gave up medical practice and began to study chemistry, which he subsidised by eeking out a modest living by writing and translating.

In 1790, while translating a textbook by the eminent Scottish physician Cullen, he came across a section dealing with the treatment of malaria by quinine. Although this was (and still is) an appropriate treatment for the disease, he was unconvinced by Cullen's explanation that it worked by virtue of having a tonic effect upon the stomach. He reasoned that since other more powerful 'tonics' had no such beneficial effect, it had to be working by some other mechanism. Accordingly, chemistry experimenter that he was, he dosed himself with quinine for several days, the result being that he began to experience the symptoms of malaria.

Thus the germ of an idea began to form – that a drug which produced the symptoms of an illness in a healthy subject could also be used to treat an illness with the same characteristics.

Over the following years Hahnemann returned to medical practice, developing the concept of *similia similibus curentur*, by dosing himself, his family and friends with different substances in order to study the symptoms produced when they were given to healthy subjects. These experiments came to be known as *provings*, from the German word *prufung*, meaning 'testing.' This culminated in the publication in 1810 of his book *The Organon of Rational Healing*. In it he set down his developing ideas for his system of homoeopathic medicine.

Initially Hahnemann prescribed his remedies in the standard dosages of the day. However, although his results were good, he found that many of his patients suffered an initial aggravation of their symptoms before receiving any benefit. In an attempt to counter this he started giving one-tenth doses. The results were good, but the aggravations, though less marked, still occurred. He therefore continued diluting the doses, each time giving a tenth of the previous dose. Predictably the aggravations disappeared, but so too did any beneficial effect. The dilutions had reached a point where there was no more medication left.

Homoeopathy might have died a death at that point had Hahnemann not discovered an incredible phenomenon. He found that by vigorously shaking each progressive dilution, the resultant remedy became not only less likely to produce aggravations, but it became more potent. This process he termed *potentisation*.

As we shall see shortly, this is one of the bedrocks of homoeopathy.

The spread of homoeopathy

By the time of Hahnemann's death at the age of 88 in 1843, homoeopathy had spread far and wide. In England, Dr Harvey Quin founded the British Homoeopathic Society in 1844 and was instrumental in opening the London Homoeopathic Hospital in 1850.

Other converts to the method carried it further afield. By the end of the 19th Century there were homoeopathic hospitals all over Europe, Russia, the two Americas and the Indian subcontinent. Indeed, at the present time there are probably more homoeopathic practitioners in India than in any other country in the world.

The Vital Force

Fundamental to Hahnemann's theory of homoeopathy was the concept of the Vital Force. He wrote:

'*Without the Vital Force the material body is unable to feel, or act, or maintain itself.*'

In his view the remedy acted not upon the disease, but upon the Vital Force to restore balance within the body.

Hahnemann was not, of course, the first to formulate the concept of Vital Force. In fact, it had been accepted for many centuries by several civilised cultures. The Ancient Chinese knew it as *Chi* and the Indian yogis called it *Prana*. In addition it has also been postulated by various individuals throughout history. For example, Paracelsus called it *Munia*, the alchemists termed it *Vital Fluid*, and Baron Von Reichenbach, the German chemist who discovered creosote, called it *Odyle*. In this century Wilhelm Reich called it *Orgone*.

In all of these cases, although there is a slightly different interpretation, it is regarded as a form of energy which permeates living creatures during life and which is an integral part of their whole being.

Orthodox Medicine does not teach this, because it is firmly

based upon a biomedical model which views the body as an intricate machine made up of a vast number of cells, each of which functions like a tiny biochemical factory. These cells are organised into tissues, the tissues into organs, and the organs into systems. Governing all of this activity is the brain, a biological computer of incredible complexity.

There is much which this model fails to explain. Life in all its myriad forms and complexities is obviously more than mere chemical reactions in cells, spurts of hormones into the blood stream and bursts of electrical nervous activity. Without even considering a spiritual dimension it is surely clear that mere chemistry cannot explain awareness, thought and the whole panoply of emotions which are part and parcel of life.

As we go up the evolutionary ladder from the simplest unicellular organisms the function of the cells which make up the organism become more specialised and less independent. With fairly complicated organisms whole groups of cells become 'tissues,' sharing a common function which other tissues cannot perform. The extreme form of this is to be found in the human nerve cells which are incapable of functioning as anything other than nerve cells because their role is so specialised.

The organisation of cells is something which the biomedical model fails to explain. Just how do cells develop into one type or another? And once they have developed into a tissue-type what makes them continue to function in a coordinated manner with their neighbours? How do the tissues manage to maintain their integrity?

It is a fact that the cells of the body are constantly dying off and being replaced. Obviously there must be a fine balance between the two, otherwise our tissues and organs would soon degenerate into complete chaos. Is it possible that the neighbouring cells have some sort of 'awareness' of the state of health of a dying cell, perhaps from the release of chemicals, or what? Some sort of control is clearly being exerted, yet the biomedical model fails to adequately explain it.

There is now a growing body of evidence which suggests that the controlling influence is not biochemical, but biophysical. Indeed, it accords well with the concept of the Vital Force of Hahnemann, taking the form of a field within and around the organism to produce a sort of *etheric body*.

In recent years biophysicists have investigated this etheric body and concluded that it is an energy field, like a plasma constellation of ionised particles. Accordingly, it has been called *biological plasma* or *bioplasma*.

Such an energy system is thought to function as an information system which acts as a template for foetal development, tissue organisation and for trouble-shooting tissue repair. It is effectively an energy double of the physical body which is intricately connected through it as a pervasive, interweaving bioelectronic network, with all the subcellular structures and organic molecules forming a semi-conductor system.

Further, because the etheric and physical bodies are so connected, each has the potential to affect the other. In terms of health the implication is that illness can arise from direct effects on either the physical or the etheric body.

As we shall see in the next chapter, our thoughts and emotions are also intimately connected with this subtle framework. And this is why homoeopathy has so much to offer.

THE PRINCIPLES OF HOMOEOPATHY

From the above brief outline it should be fairly clear that apart from the existence of the Vital Force, the two main principles of homoeopathy are the Law of Similars and the use of potentised remedies. Let us now look at them in a little more detail.

The Law of Similars

This means that a substance which produces symptoms of a disease in a well person can also be used to treat someone who has that disease. Hence, *similia similibus curentur* – let like be treated by like.

Effectively one takes the symptom-complex of the patient and attempts to match it up with the toxic effect-complex of the remedy. There may be several remedies which are close, but the nearest match is the 'similar.' As an example, belladonna poisoning causes a toxic effect-complex which resembles the disease of scarlet fever. If someone suffering with scarlet fever presents in the classic manner, then belladonna would be the appropriate similar.

This is a fairly clear cut case. It is important to appreciate, however, that in homoeopathy one is trying to match the remedy profile to the patient profile, not to the disease profile. To explain this, consider five men of similar age and background, who all complain of feeling depressed. The same orthodox medication, a tricyclic antidepressant may be appropriate for all five. A homoeopath, however, would look at the symptom patterns of each individual and could well end up prescribing a completely different remedy for each man. It is, after all, the individual that is being treated homoeopathically, not the disease.

The Law of Cure

Another important homoeopathic principle is the Law of Cure, formulated by an American homoeopath, Constantine Hering. It states that a cure is effected:

from above downwards
from within outwards
from major to lesser organs
and it takes place in reverse order of appearance
of the symptoms.

Thus, one starts to feel emotionally better before physical improvement comes. Similarly, with an illness which presented with a cough then a rash, the rash (being last to come) would disappear before the cough settled.

Remedies from many sources

The modern homoeopathic materia medica contains well over two thousand remedies. All sorts of things are used, from simple things like common salt, to exotic cacti, snake venom and precious metals like gold.

In the treatment of emotional problems we use those substances which, if taken in their pure form can induce particular emotions or feelings in well people. For example, the poison arsenic makes individuals very anxious; sepia (cuttle-fish ink) induces depressed mood; strychnine causes irritability and anger.

Potency and the infinitesimal dose

Although homoeopathy is associated with using infinitesimal amounts of substances, it is the Law of Similars which is the crux of the method. If the incorrect remedy is chosen the question of potency is almost irrelevant.

Potency means far more than dilution. The process of potentisation actually seems to enhance the 'power' of a remedy, so that it becomes more potent. The remedy becomes less concentrated but more energised.

In order to prepare homoeopathic medicines two methods are used. Firstly, for soluble substances an alcoholic extract is made by infusion for up to three weeks, followed by filtration to produce a *mother tincture*. This is then diluted with 40 per cent alcohol to one in ten or one in a hundred. This is then vigorously vibrated for a few seconds, a process called *succussion*, to produce the first potency remedy on the two commonest potency scales.

The 1:10 scale is called the *Decimal scale* and is designated by the letter 'X' in the UK, and by 'D' on the continent. Thus the first potency would be 1X.

The 1:100 scale is called the *Centesimal scale* and is designated by the letter 'C' in the UK, and by 'CH' on the continent. Thus the first potency would be 1C.

To prepare the next potency one part of the first potency would be taken and diluted 1:10 or 1:100, then succussed as before to produce the 2X or 2C potencies.

It will now be very clear that it does not take many dilutions to dramatically reduce the concentration of a substance. By the 6th process on the decimal scale (6X), which is the equivalent of the 3rd on the centesimal scale (3C), the mother tincture will be diluted to one in a million. By the 6th process on the centesimal scale (6C) the dilution will be one in a billion. These figures are quite incredible. Indeed, according to Avogadro's Law, by the time one reaches 12C the solution is unlikely to have even a single molecule of the original compound left.

The second method is for insoluble substances which cannot be made into mother tinctures. In this case they are mechanically ground together with lactose powder for several hours in the proportion of one in ten, a process called *trituration*. This process is repeated three times to produce a 3X potency, after which it can be dissolved in alcohol and water, then potentised in the usual manner.

By convention, 12C is the cut off point, all remedies up to this being considered low potency and those of 12C and above being high potency.

How do the remedies work?
From what we have just seen about the potencies it is clear that only the low potencies can possibly work in the accepted pharmacological sense through a chemical reaction. Once one exceeds Avogadro's number, which happens at 12C, there cannot logically be any of the original remedy left in the solution. If the remedies still work, which they decidedly do, then they clearly must be working in some other more subtle manner. Rather than working biochemically, I believe that they are working biophysically.

Research carried out over the past forty or so years has looked at the potency question. Studies on enzymes, the growth of yeasts and seedlings have all demonstrated that appropriate homoeopathic preparations exert an effect even when one has gone past the Avogadro level of 12C.

Curiously, however, it is an observed phenomenon that the effect under study seems to wax and wane with succeeding potency levels. For example, when measuring the effect of a homoeopathic substance on the growth of wheat seedlings a boosting effect may appear at 7C, followed by a retarding effect at 9C, then a boosting effect at 11C. The actual magnitude of the boost may be no more at 11C than at 7C, as indeed, the retarding effect may be the same at 9C, 13C and 17C. This suggests that they are working in an energetic wave-form manner.

One of the most celebrated pieces of research in recent years was that published by Professor Jaques Benveniste of Paris, in the scientific journal *Nature* in June 1988. He reported upon the ability of 'homoeopathically prepared' (my parenthesis) dilutions of Anti-IgE in the range up to 60C to cause particular types of white blood cell to lose their staining ability. Like previous workers he discovered a wave-like effect of activity and inactivity with successive potentisations.

These studies were repeated and confirmed in five other laboratories throughout the world – another in France, two in Israel, one in Italy and one in Canada.

One of Benveniste's conclusions was that since dilutions need to be accompanied by vigorous shaking for the effects to be observed, transmission of the biological information could be related to the molecular organisation of the water. In other words, the water somehow retains an energetic imprint of the original molecule's

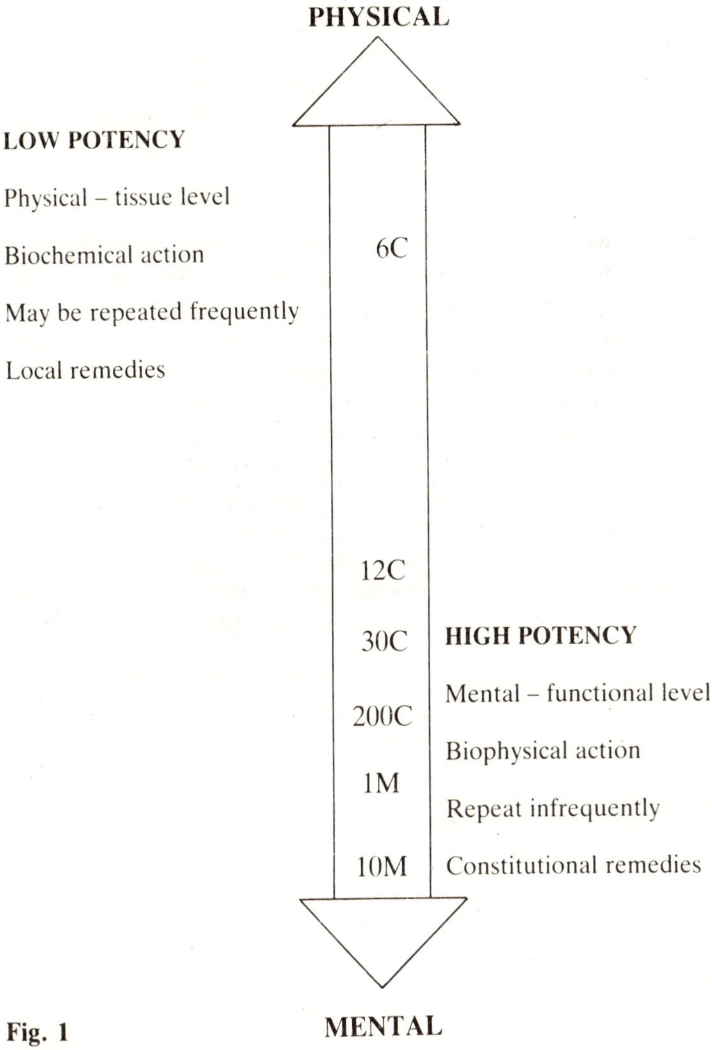

Fig. 1

energy, perhaps retained in the way molecules of water connect to one another through their hydrogen bonding.

And this brings us to the nature of the remedy itself. It is not the chemistry of the compound used to make the remedy that matters, but its very energy, its *vibrational pattern*. It is the fact that it 'vibrates' in the similar manner to the 'vibration' of the individual's illness state, or to the pattern he presents to the world through his symptoms, signs, feelings and attitudes. When he takes the remedy, it is the remedy's vibration which stimulates the etheric body to reharmonise itself, resulting in the ultimate rebalancing of the physical body.

Which potency?

Within the world of homoeopathy there is considerable debate as to whether it is best to use low or high potency. My own opinion is that it depends upon what one is trying to do. I believe that with problems which are most obviously rooted in the physical body the low potencies are most appropriate, since they have more of a biochemical, tissue level effect. On the other hand, where a problem is 'emotional' or causing an 'emotional problem,' there is more need to aim the treatment at the etheric body. Thus, since there is more of a need to work at the biophysical range, one should use the higher potencies. (Fig. 1 on previous page.)

For the above reasons I RECOMMEND THE 30C or 200C POTENCIES FOR ALL PROBLEMS COVERED IN THIS BOOK (See the section on 'taking the remedies' at the beginning of Part 3).

CHAPTER 3

The Importance of Emotions in Homoeopathy

> *Thus, behind all disease lie our fears, our anxieties, our greed, our likes and our dislikes. Let us seek these out and heal them, and with the healing of them will go the disease from which we suffer.*
>
> Dr Edward Bach, *The Twelve Healers*

The Law of Similars is the bedrock of homoeopathy. The similar, the best possible match of remedy-complex to patient-complex, will yield the best chance of successful treatment.

In the last chapter we looked at the way the remedy might work upon the individual through effects on the etheric and physical bodies. It is because the energetic nature of the remedy metaphorically 'vibrates' in the same way as the overall picture of the individual in his ill or 'dis-eased' state, that it causes a reharmonisation. In other words it induces the individual's Vital Force to begin self-healing.

Maya, the world of illusion

There is a concept in Hindu philosophy which states that we exist in a world of illusion, called *maya*. Although this was very much a philosophical conclusion, quantum physics has given us scientific insights into this Ancient wisdom.

All matter is made up of molecules and all molecules are made up of atoms, which in turn are made up of subatomic particles.

Nothing, absolutely nothing in our physical world is at rest. It vibrates, it has energy and *it is energy*.

The human body is made up of cells, tissues, organs and organ systems. If one thinks of the motion of each subatomic particle, each atom, each molecule within that incredibly complicated structure then it is clear that a phenomenal amount of activity is going on. Not only is there the functioning of the physical body, but there is the activity of the mind in thought and the perception of its emotional state.

As we discussed earlier, the etheric body and the physical body are not separate entities, but are intricately connected. Each is affected by the other, so that dysfunction in one can affect the other. The etheric body represents the energetic side of existence, the physical body the material side.

And this is where we come to the concept of *maya*, the illusion of reality. While all things are in movement, are energetic and are a form of energy, we perceive them through the senses of our physical body as being other than they are. In other words we are limited in what we perceive by virtue of the limitations of our five senses. For example we see only within a narrow band of the electromagnetic spectrum. We hear a very limited range of sounds, and we can only physically feel objects which have a particular level of substantiality – although we are surrounded by gases, we do not 'feel them'. True, we have tools and technology which can help us to 'see', 'hear' and 'touch' beyond the range of our senses, yet even then the tools and technology are restricted in their level of function.

The underlying reality is far more complicated than the illusion would have us believe.

Tapping into the individual's vibration

In the light of what we have just discussed it should be clear that all individuals have a 'vibration' which is unique to them. It is a composite of their body and etheric functions, their thoughts, perceptions and emotions. The whole aim of homoeopathy is to tune into this vibration in order to deduce which remedy will best restore balance.

The homoeopathic diagnostic process aims at accumulating as much information as possible about the individual's experience of existence. Effectively, this allows one to interpret the individual's vibration.

Heart and Soul

In assessing the correct remedy it is necessary to work out what is important in the individual's history. Of prime importance here is a knowledge about the individual's *mental and emotional symptoms*. This means paying particular attention to the *likes and dislikes, hates and passions, fears, anxieties, dreams and aspirations*.

To use an older expression one attempts to look at the contents of the heart and soul of the individual.

For example, is there a liking for some quality in life? Is it an admiration, an obsession which one must follow, or a fanatacism which completely dominates one's life? Does frustration in that line lead to anger, despair, jealousy or some other emotion?

Also of marked importance is the 'nature' of the individual. Is he or she generally optimistic, pessimistic, placcid, aggressive, domineering, flexible, inflexible, and so on? Is the image they project to the world, what Jung called *the persona*, a true reflection of what the individual feels, or is it merely a facade?

And again, what are the memories which the individual stores up? Is he obsessed with past slights and grievances, does he only see the best in others, does he care what happens to those about him?

All of these are vitally important in assessing the correct remedy. And this holds true for all situations, not merely when using homoeopathy for emotional problems.

The gradation of symptoms

As mentioned above, the mental and emotional symptoms are of the greatest importance in remedy selection. There are other *general symptoms*, which while having lesser significance, can lead one to choose the similar.

Thus, in looking for a remedy the symptoms should be looked at according to the following gradation of importance:

the mental and emotional symptoms – the emotional make-up, psychological tendencies; whether better for such things as consolation, music, stress; introversion or extroversion; fears; sex drive etc.

the modalities – those things or factors which make the individual feel better or worse. Being indoors or outdoors; weather preferences; times of day; preference for movement etc.

likes and dislikes – foods and drinks; craving for such things as salt.

physical features – certain physical features, outlooks, manners may be very relevant.

As we shall also see, there may be particular physical diseases and emotional problems which may be additional pointers to the choice of remedy. Thus:

disease tendencies – the conditions to which one is prone. These may have been problems in the past, but have 'burned out.'

emotional tendencies – the emotional problems to which the individual is prone. For example, a tendency to problems associated with fear, anger, jealousy, guilt, etc.

In addition, there may be *particular symptoms* associated with a remedy which make it quite characteristic.

The above framework is the one which shall be used throughout the Materia Medica of this book.

Emotions and the Law of Cure

To recap on this homoeopathic principle, cure tends to occur *from above downwards*

from within outwards
from major to lesser organs
and it takes place in reverse order of
appearance of the symptoms

The significance of this is that if the correct remedy is chosen, the emotional problems will tend to improve first, since the 'mind' is the highest realm, and because it reflects the activity of the brain which is the most important organ. However, if the emotional problem developed last, for example after a prolonged physical illness, then it would take time to go.

Aggravation of symptoms

Homoeopathic remedies often produce a temporary aggravation of symptoms as they start to work. When using them in acute conditions the aggravation is usually short-lived, whereas in a more chronic condition it may last for a few days. Following this one usually finds that the condition starts to improve.

If there has been suppression of emotional symptoms in the past, then as the Vital Force starts the healing process those suppressed emotions may recur for a short time. These represent unblocking of pent-up energies and are, in fact, a good sign.

In addition to this, however, an appropriately chosen remedy may cause other physical signs to become manifest after some time. For example, if there has been eczema or asthma in the past, then this may flare-up for a short period.

And finally, in some people a 'healing crisis' may develop after a week or two. Here there may be worsening of the condition and the symptoms of a cold, or tummy bug may seem to come on. Again, it should only last for a day or two.

Some Cases

Let us now look at a few examples.

Miss R.W., aged 17 years, a prefect at a girl's high school. Had always been popular and was often chosen to demonstrate things in class. Seemed to be extroverted, yet secretly agonised about such things for days beforehand. When she was told that she would have to read the morning lesson at assembly, she became extremely apprehensive and developed a diarrhoeal illness two weeks before the scheduled event. She consulted, asking for 'something to calm her down.'

She was prescribed Argentum nitricum with an excellent result. The anticipatory anxiety disappeared, as did the diarrhoea. She performed excellently on the morning of the assembly and actually enjoyed the experience.

Mrs P.B., aged 43 years, a housewife and mother of three. Her problems started after a dinner party given by a colleague of her husband's after he had gained a senior management post in a national organisation. She began to feel depressed, irritable and extremely jealous. She became preoccupied with the thought that he was being unfaithful to her. It started to take over her life. She checked his pockets, his case and his car for any evidence of him having an affair with another woman.

She had always tended to be a chatterbox, but now her conversation became dominated by her feelings of jealousy. Also, her temper had always been short just before a period, but now the tantrums started coming more frequently. On several occasions she struck out at her husband. She was aware that the children were being affected by her moods.

She consulted when she realised that her marriage was getting into a precarious condition. She was diagnosed as needing Lachesis, which she took after her menstrual periods over three months. The jealousy improved straight away, followed by the irritability and the depression.

Mr J.D., aged 55 years, an electrician. After sustaining a severe electrical burn while carrying out re-wiring work in a factory, he developed a marked anxiety state. This was followed by a need to check common things in the home. He was unable to leave any appliance plugged in and had to ensure that the removed plug was placed exactly one foot from the socket. So intense did this compulsive behaviour become that he felt unable to leave the house. Unplugging the television set, for example, would take about an hour, because of the precision with which he made himself arrange the plug and the wires.

He had always been a meticulous workman. Everything about him was neat and ordered. Everything had a place.

He was prescribed Aconite at first, which started to help with the generalised anxiety. This was followed by Arsenicum album. Over the following six months his obsessive-compulsive behaviour disappeared.

Mrs E.E., aged 63 years, a retired nurse who had tended to her husband over a final illness. After his death she found herself unable to weep or grieve. Two months later she developed severe migraine and literally 'drew up the drawbridge.' She cut herself off from her friends and relatives and became a virtual recluse. Pressure from a worried niece forced her to accept medical aid.

She had lost her appetite for most things. She rarely cooked a proper meal, coming to depend upon her frying pan. Bacon sandwiches became her staple food. In addition, she was going through an excessive quantity of paracetamol a day.

She was thought to need Natrum muriaticum. After one treatment she experienced a flood of tears, a lifting of her depressed mood and a relief from the headaches. Two more treatments over the next few weeks brought about an improvement in her confidence and she started to socialise again.

Dr K.A., aged 27 years, a young hospital doctor specialising in neurosurgery. She suddenly lost her enthusiasm for surgery, her career and her fiance. She became indifferent to everyone around her, lost interest in her studies (she was preparing for a higher surgical qualification) and lost enthusiasm for playing hockey, a sport at which she excelled.

She had attributed her low spirits and indifference to a reactive depression brought on by having to deal with several particularly traumatic neurosurgical cases.

She was diagnosed as needing Sepia, which she was given after her next three menstrual periods. Her improvement was dramatic.

Homoeopathy, a logical choice for emotional problems

Emotions are part of life. Virtually everyone experiences at some time or another the whole range of emotions. Without them life would be very dull. For some people, however, they are so affected that life or part of it becomes a trial, a drudge, or even abject misery. Homoeopathy, since it primarily focuses on the individual's mental and emotional symptoms, offers an ideal and logical means of calming the troubled waters of the mind.

CHAPTER 4

Vulnerable Constitutions

Study the patient not the disease

James Tyler Kent

Throughout history it has been a basic aim of many medical systems to identify 'types' of people. In particular, the desire has been to link up emotional profiles, physical characteristics, strengths and weaknesses in order to work out in what way the individual's internal balance is impaired so that the treatment can be tailored to meet his needs.

According to Ayurvedic Medicine, which is practised extensively throughout India, there are three humours, or vital energies or fluids, which can join together in various combinations at a person's birth. These combinations result in the production of seven constitutional types. Essentially, the Ayurvedic physician aims to determine the individual constitution and treat it appropriately.

Islamic Medicine, which is based upon the teachings of Hippocrates and Galen, also has a humoral theory. Like Ayurveda it proposes that the humours combine together at birth to form a basic constitutional type. And since there are four humours in this system the number of constitutional types is extended to eleven.

The constitution in homoeopathy

In homoeopathy we recognise the concept of the constitutional type. By this we mean the combination of psychological and physical features of the person, together with the way they interact with and react to their environment.

These constitutional types are described in terms of the remedy profile which most closely suits the personality and overall profile of that individual. Thus a homoeopath might talk about an 'Arsenicum type,' or a 'Phosphorus' or a 'Sulphur type.'

One thing should be made clear, however, and that is that there are very many different constitutional types of remedies, since each person is an individual. In homoeopathy we make no attempt to categorise people into a set number of categories, as is done in Ayurvedic Medicine and Unani Medicine. Simply, we try to match up the person profile to the remedy profile.

Characteristic emotional features

Some remedies have very marked emotional aspects which make selection relatively simple.

These include:-

the fear of *Aconite*
the despair and suicidal thoughts of *Aurum metallicum*
the anticipatory nervousness of *Argentum nitricum*
the obsessive fussiness and tidiness of *Arsenicum album*
the slowness and depression of *Calcarea carbonica*
the restless irritability of *Chamomilla*
the capriciousness and moodiness of *Ignatia*
the jealousy of *Lachesis*
the anger and irritability of *Nux vomica*
the pride and arrogance of *Platina*
the tearfulness and changeable symptoms of *Pulsatilla*
the indifference of *Sepia*

Vulnerable constitutions

From a look at the above examples it should be clear that certain constitutional types are liable to fall victim to certain emotional problems.

Let us now look at a few examples.

Argentum Nitricum

Key features: anticipatory anxiety, constant hurry, impulsive, claustrophobia, tormented by troublesome thoughts, 'brain fag.'

These types are nervous, tremulous and impulsive.

From their earliest days Argentum nitricum people will be in a hurry. As children they will want things to move. They will want other people to move quickly and they will tend to walk fast so that people have to keep up with them.

As children they may have a problem with bed-wetting.

While they are not timid, they develop anticipatory anxiety. They will agree to do things, feel pleased to take them on, yet agonise for days, even weeks before the event. It is likely to affect their bowels to cause loose diarrhoea.

They may become high achievers, partly because they fear failure so much.

Enclosed spaces are a source of dread for them. In childhood they will shy away from tunnels, caves and cupboards. In adulthood this may extend to lifts, small rooms and crowded places. They may anticipate the worst possible situation and always ensure that they have a quick means of exit so as to prevent getting trapped. In a cinema or theatre they will try to get the end seat in the row, at a football match they will try to get a place near the exit.

They have a tendency to get troublesome thoughts which are hard to get rid of. Often these are to do with their own health. For example, there may be a fear that they are going to be sick in a certain situation. They may fear that they will faint, that their heart will stop, or that their mental faculties are progressively failing.

These troublesome thoughts can torment them. Sometimes they are quite irrational and make them do strange impulsive things. A youngster on a bicycle may find that he cannot turn right, because he does not feel able to turn his head to the right at the same time as sticking the right arm out. Consequently, he will tend to plot a course which allows him to take the fewest number of right turns.

Adults might similarly have troublesome thoughts associated with high buildings, cliffs and bridges. They may feel impelled to jump off, so they may avoid the situation. This could develop into an apparent phobia, although it is more likely to be the fear of the Lemming impulse which keeps them away, rather than the fear of physical injury. Curiously, the tendency to walk faster and faster may be caused by some such fear of someone or something stalking them.

They may be embarrassed by these peculiar reasons for their impulsive actions or apparent phobias, so they will not talk about them.

Mental activity may make them quite exhausted and they may get 'brain fag.' The student about to take an exam may suffer the characteristic Argentum nitricum anticipatory anxiety with looseness of the motions, then get a feeling of the knowledge suddenly 'going.' This might heighten the anxiety to produce tremulousness and palpitations.

Headaches are commonly associated with coldness and trembling. Strong emotional upsets may provoke a headache or a migraine. Tight pressure will often relieve it.

Physical symptoms are generally worse for heat and for concentration. They are better not thinking about their problems.

Splinter-like sensations are common, especially in the throat. Indeed, most pains will have some splinter-like quality to them.

They may develop cravings for chocolate and sweet things. Indeed, there may be a tendency to overeat, possibly culminating in the development of a bulimia problem.

Arsenicum Album

Key features: anguish, anxiety, restlessness, obsessiveness, regular recurrences, over-sensitiveness, agitated depression.

These individuals are quick, restless, neat and extremely tidy.

As children they stand out because they are so neat. While other children throw things all around them, leaving rooms in disorder, the Arsenicum album types carefully fold, stack and put away in order. They dislike being dirty and will insist upon being clean. Even the baby unable to talk will let it be known that they are not prepared to sit in a damp and soiled nappy.

As they get a little bit older their sense of aesthetics develops. They like pretty and beautiful things which they can collect, organise and categorise.

But as they get older they also get fussy and nervous. They fuss and bother about other people. They organise the family, make appointments for them and get bothered if their efforts are not heeded.

They get upset if things are left lying around. They feel that everything has its place and they will try to ensure that there is a place for everything. Books have to be in neat rows, magazines have to be stacked and symmetry is regarded as an ideal. Dusting must not be skimped upon and the house is always kept clean.

They are over-sensitive in every way. Any illness seems the worst it can possibly be. Any pain really 'burns.' Surprisingly, rather than being helped by coolness the burning is improved by heat and warmth.

They dislike strong smells, strong tastes and bright light. On the other hand, they also dislike the dark – but because of a fear of what might be lurking there. Indeed, they will always sleep well wrapped up, without even a toe protruding from the covers, although they rarely like the head to be covered.

They may fear many things, especially if it involves some unknown factor, eg the dark, burglars, ghosts, death, illness.

They can readily sink into a depression. They will be restless, unable to settle and they will fidget.

They may develop habit problems and they may drink too much. The old lady with her neat home and sherry bottle at the ready is a classic example.

Their physical problems may tend to recur at regular or periodic intervals and they tend to suffer from aggravations round about midnight.

Looseness is another feature. They get loose runny noses with colds; loose coughs and asthma; loose diarrhoea and vomiting.

In general they tend to be thirsty, but prefer to drink small quantities frequently.

Calcarea Carbonica

Key features: Lethargic depression, fears, slowness, congestion, chronic fatigue, jealousy and hate.

This constitutional type seems to go through definite phases, or potential problem periods as they get older.

The Calcarea carbonica individual tends to be flabby, easily moved to depression and with generalised slowness of both movement and thought.

As a toddler they are slow to produce teeth, but the gums get raw, swollen and painful as the arrival is awaited. With each tooth they seem to get 'teething problems.' They get teething coughs, rashes and bouts of vomiting sour milk.

As they get a bit older they get podgy and like to be left alone. You can sit the Calcarea carbonica toddler down and he will not charge around, he will sit, and watch and wait.

In adulthood the podginess may go, yet there will still be a flabby appearance to the face, the neck perhaps seeming slightly thin in proportion. More usually though, the appearance is of a fair, fat, flabby type of person. The handgrip is loose, the energy is low. They will tend to perspire, mainly over the head and chest, even when it isn't hot. They will tire easily, complain of breathlessness and may get bloating in the abdomen.

Anaemia, gall stones, period problems, warts, cramps of all sorts and swelling of the glands with any infection. All this is she prone to.

In middle age we find the tendency to develop chronic catarrh and chest problems.

In older age the above problems are all compounded by all sorts of congestion, including congestive cardiac failure, chronic obstructive airways disease and chronic constipation. Added to this is the tendency to develop back pains, again reflecting the problem with calcification in the supporting tissue of the body.

And there are fears. All sorts of fear, from impending doom, to developing insanity and even death.

All types of exertion, be it mental or physical, tend to exhaust Calcarea carbonica types. This does not mean that they cannot cope, they assuredly can, but it may be at a price.

They may be prone to develop a Chronic Fatigue Syndrome.

Because they are lethargic and slow, they may find themselves being compared unfavourably with others who seem to be more vivacious and dynamic. As a result they may suffer jealousy. Sometimes it can become actual hatred.

In general they hate the open air, dislike outdoor pursuits and get 'chilled' easily.

Early in life they generally love eggs above all other foods, although they are partial to ice cream, sweets, raw vegetables and 'curious tastes' like chalky mixtures. Milk, on the other hand makes them worse. It disagrees with them, from the vomiting of sour milk as a baby to the nausea of milk and milk products advised for the flatulence of adulthood.

Nux Vomica

Key features: anxious, fiery, irritability, easily-offended, over-sensitive, melancholic, fastidious, tendency to use stimulants, habituation, insomnia.

This constitutional type will always present a fiery, slightly tetchy front to the world. The child will know what it wants and at times make it known that they want it.

As they get older the temper will become apparent. They will argue and quarrel, possibly making good debators. When things are going badly, however, they will dislike being contradicted. As a result they may become quite irritable and fly off into a rage.

When they are frustrated over trifles they may respond in an exaggerated manner. If they have been painstakingly putting a model together, but the finishing stages prove extra tricky, or if things go slightly wrong, they may destroy the whole thing. An essay might end up crumpled in a ball if it is criticised. A chair in their way may be kicked over. At times they might even hit out at other people.

In general, however, they tend to be fastidious and neat. They often take lots of things on, possibly becoming very successful in business. But with the success comes the anxiety. While they can keep their affairs in order all will be well, but there is a tendency to take too much on. They dislike delegating things, so that they end up attending to everything. It is the attention to the smallest matters which is likely to upset them most.

Insomnia is common because of the preoccupation with business. They may wake about 3am, the affairs of business immediately flooding into the mind.

They can become depressed when things or events overwhelm them. When they do, they tend to be quite agitated in their depression.

In order to cope they may seek the aid of stimulants. Tobacco, coffee, alcohol and drugs, they may all be resorted to in excess. Indeed, too much of any of them, or to much rich food may well induce a hangover effect. It would consist of a dull headache, worse for moving the eyes, and a gastritis. There may well be nausea. With the hangover, of course, would come the typical irritability and the over-sensitivity.

This over-sensitivity covers the whole range, from criticism and casual comments, to distaste for noise, smells and, when unwell, movement.

There is a marked sensitivity to dry winds. When there is a sudden change in the weather with such a wind, they may develop a headache, become irritable, fiery and even physically aggressive.

Constipation may trouble them, with difficulty in straining. Similarly, the passage of urine may require straining with poor result.

Sepia

Key features: Indifference, depression, weepiness, dislike of sympathy, very negative, resentful, better for exertion, hypochondriasis and Chronic Fatigue Syndrome.

This constitutional type tends to have bouts of lack of interest. Even as a child they may become sluggish, lose interest in toys and play. If cajoled into action which they do not want, they are likely to cry or start sulking.

They seem to become depressed particularly easily. They hate being touched, feel worse for sympathy, yet do not like to be left on their own.

When they are particularly depressed or under pressure they feel indifferent to others. Even their closest friends and relatives hold little interest for them. They wish they could be left alone (even though they hate being alone), and they feel like just running away.

In talking about their problems they tend to weep. Indeed, weeping often helps, because they feel better for a 'good cry.'

Fears may spring up. They may fear poverty, losing their mind, or of developing some incurable chronic disease.

Music may make them cry, but curiously, dancing has an almost magical effect. The indifferent, gloomy, depressed adult can suddenly come alive on the dance floor.

Resentment is common. They may feel wounded by simple slights, feel resentment for neighbours or friends who try to help, and they may hold grudges for years.

The periods may be very heavy and accompanied by a marked dragging-down sensation. Premenstrual problems are common. Similarly, they often find the menopause a difficult time of life.

* * *

From these five examples you can see how the basic nature of a constitution can predispose them to certain types of emotional problems. When faced with stress they tend to react to it according to their constitution, so that the manifestation of that stress could be to develop an anxiety state (eg, Arsenicum album), a phobic state (eg, Argentum nitricum), a depression (eg Calcarea carbonicum), a drug dependence or alcohol problem (eg Nux vomica), or a state of withdrawal (eg Sepia.)

This is not to say that Argentum nitricum is the remedy to be thought of when faced by a phobia, nor is Nux vomica the remedy for a drug dependency. No, that would be an over-simplified and misleading concept. What is implied is that while some constitutions are vulnerable to particular emotions and emotional problems, the way they experience them is characteristic of that constitution. For example, Arsenicum album, Calcarea carbonica and Sepia types can all become depressed, but the manner in which they feel depressed and the way in which they react will be quite different.

This is the difference between orthodox medicine and homoeopathy. Whereas a single antidepressant drug could be given to all three types to treat *the* depression, in homoeopathy the *similar remedy* would have to be given to the patient according to the symptom pattern in order to treat *the* patient.

Vulnerable Constitutions

The following constitutional remedies are generally vulnerable to the following types of emotional problems (Details will, of course, be found under the appropriate chapters):-

Panic attacks
Gelsemium
Kali phosphoricum

General fearful conditions
Argentum nitricum
Arsenicum album
Calcarea carbonica
Causticum
Gelsemium
Kali phosphoricum
Lycopodium
Natrum muriaticum
Phosphorus
Pulsatilla
Sulphur

Phobias
Argentum nitricum
Arsenicum album
Calcarea carbonica
Causticum
Gelsemium
Lachesis
Lycopodium
Mercurius solubilis
Natrum muriaticum
Nux vomica
Phosphorus
Pulsatilla
Sulphur

Fixations, obsessions or compulsions
Argentum nitricum
Arsenicum album
Ignatia
Lachesis
Phosphorus

Fixations, obsessions or compulsions
Pulsatilla
Sepia
Silica
Sulphur

Sadness and depression
Arsenicum album
Calcarea carbonica
Graphites
Ignatia
Kali phosphoricum
Natrum muriaticum
Nitricum acidum
Nux vomica
Phosphorus
Pulsatilla
Sepia
Sulphur

Guilt
Arsenicum album
Causticum
Graphites
Ignatia
Natrum muriaticum
Nitricum acidum
Nux vomica
Pulsatilla

Love-sickness
Causticum
Ignatia
Lachesis
Natrum muriaticum
Nux vomica
Sepia

Hate
Calcarea carbonica
Lachesis
Natrum muriaticum
Nitricum acidum
Phosphorus

Jealousy
Arsenicum album
Calcarea carbonica
Ignatia
Lachesis
Lycopodium
Nux vomica
Pulsatilla

Irritability and anger
Arsenicum album
Hepar sulph
Ignatia
Lachesis
Lycopodium
Natrum muriaticum
Nitricum acidum
Nux vomica
Phosphorus
Pulsatilla
Sepia
Sulphur

Grief
Arsenicum album
Causticum
Ignatia
Lachesis
Natrum muriaticum
Pulsatilla
Sepia

Exhaustion and chronic fatigue
Calcarea carbonica
Kali phosphoricum
Lycopodium
Mercurius solubilis
Sepia

Insomnia
Arsenicum album
Ignatia
Kali phosphoricum
Nux vomica
Phosphorus
Sulphur

Eating disorders
Argentum nitricum
Calcarea carbonica
Causticum
Graphites
Natrum muriaticum
Phosphorus
Pulsatilla
Sulphur

Premenstrual syndrome
Lachesis
Natrum muriaticum
Sepia

Habituations and dependencies
Arsenicum album
Argentum nitricum
Ignatia
Lachesis
Nux vomica
Sulphur

CHAPTER 5

Mixed Emotions and Coping

Poetry is the spontaneous overflow of powerful feelings: it takes its origin from emotion recollected in tranquillity.

William Wordsworth, *Lyrical Ballads*

Tranquillity, the state of calmness and serenity, is a pleasant base from which to write poetry. As Wordsworth implies, however, it is very much the calm after the storm. It comes after the troubled emotions have passed.

Sadly, for some people a tranquil mind is little more than a wishful dream. They may become so psychologically scarred that they seem to pass their lives in a perpetual emotional storm. One trauma may follow another to produce a state of mixed emotions.

Psychological defence mechanisms

According to psychodynamic theory, the *unconscious* constantly strives to protect the *conscious* mind from the effects of emotions such as *guilt*, by operating a series of defence mechanisms. Effectively, these unconscious mechanisms push the unwanted emotions into the unconscious part of the mind, where they do least harm!

Or least harm in the short term, that is.

Let us look at a few examples.

Denial This is one of the commonest of mechanisms. A painful or disagreeable thought or emotion is simply denied or rejected. For example, in the acute stage of grief a bereaved person feels shocked and mentally numbed, so that they simply will not accept the painful news. Indeed, up to 40 per cent of bereaved people still feel the presence of the departed loved one, and about 15 per cent frequently 'see' or 'hear' their lost one. It would seem that this unconscious denial of the facts eases the pain of the reality.

Effectively, by denying an unpleasant or unpalatable thing, there is no unpleasant reaction to deal with.

Projection This means that the blame for something is put onto someone or something else. It is the workman blaming his tools, the aggressor blaming his protagonist for being aggressive and starting the fight. One's own hostile or unpleasant feelings are projected onto another person, thereby 'justifying' the individual for reacting in the same way.

Displacement This is the deflection of feelings about one individual onto another. Thus, rather than standing up to an authority figure one may go home and kick the cat.

Some people seem to internalise with this mechanism. For example, rather than being aggressive to the person they really want to be aggressive to, they displace the feeling onto themselves. The result may be self-destructive or suicidal behaviour.

Isolation This means isolating a thought from an emotion and effectively burying the emotional feeling in the unconscious. The individual may then be able for a time to think the thought without feeling the emotion. For example, 'I hate her,' may be said without feeling the emotion of hate.

Sublimation This is a common mechanism. Aggressive or anti-social feelings may be sublimated, or channeled into some 'acceptable' form of activity, such as a contact sport.

Repression This comes about when a thought or memory is so painful that it cannot be tolerated. Accordingly, it is 'forgotten' forever, or pushed so deeply that it cannot be recalled.

Rationalisation This takes place when a logical reason can be made to excuse a feeling or thought. For example, 'I cannot afford to go to see that relative, in case he makes me lose my temper.' This is a rationalisation of the actual feeling – 'I feel angry at (the relative) and know that I will be violent towards him.'

Conversion This refers to the hysterical production of physical symptoms in order to solve an emotional conflict. For example, fear about playing an important football match could result in a physical ankle pain and limp which would allow the individual to miss the event without exhibiting the fear.

Mixed Emotions

All of the above mechanisms are unconscious means of coping with emotions which are considered 'bad' by the individual's *conscience*. By making the unpalatable thought non-threatening, by sinking the associated emotion into the unconscious, the individual is able to function normally.

However, sinking the emotion does not necessarily remove it. Very often it 'simmers' away in the depths of the unconscious, occasionally producing symptoms as 'bubbles' break the surface into the conscious mind. It is as if the emotion can only be held in check in the unconscious for so long before it needs to 'understand' why it is there. However, because the defence mechanism has effectively disconnected the thought from the emotion, it bursts into the conscious mind and produces symptoms which the conscious cannot explain.

Not only that, but very often one emotion drifts into another to produce a veritable tangle of problems. A sort of 'blockage' may form whereby the emotions cannot be released, but go on producing symptoms as ever-increasing emotional bubbles break through into the conscious mind.

Consider a young man who falls in *love* with a young woman. She spurns his advances and forms a relationship with his best friend. He becomes *jealous* of the friend, and *angry* at both of them. He starts to feel *hate* and feels *aggressive*. In his worst moments he feels as if he would like to kill them.

By operating several of the defence mechanisms his conscience allows him to 'come to terms' with the situation. That is only on the surface, however. In his unconscious the jealousy and hate bubble away. A guilt feeling starts to materialise. He begins to feel anxious. He starts to experience various unusual physical symptoms. And he feels bouts of guilt.

He starts to develop a *fixed idea*, and feels *compelled* to check things. He then builds up an elaborate superstitious ritual about knives and sharp objects, being unable to leave them alone without first touching them seven times.

This young man has thus developed a *fixation*, an obsessive-compulsive neurosis about sharp objects. He is anxious around sharp things, like knives, scissors and needles, but he is unaware as to why.

In psychodynamic terms he has developed the problem by *isolating* his emotions, and in order to undo his guilt feelings about his hate, jealousy and thoughts of violence towards the couple who were so much part of his life, he has built up this superstitious distorted guilt-ridding ritual. Unfortunately, the price is that his life has become governed by the fear and the fixation.

This is a very simplistic mixed emotion picture. We see how the emotions in the unconscious have somehow worked into a tangle to produce some sort of 'blockage' to produce the emotional problem and the fixation.

I believe that people use these mechanisms all the time. I also believe, however, that people tend to use some more frequently than others. They are geared to do so by their individual nature, by their constitutional type. Similarly, the type of emotions they experience and the ones they experience problems with, are also consequent upon their natures.

Homoeopathy and mixed emotions

In Chapter 3 we considered the individual as a composite of the physical and etheric bodies. All traumas, be they physical injuries, past infections or emotional 'blows' have an effect upon the 'vibration' of the whole person.

These problems can be compared to the build up of layers of a pearl or an onion, each layer representing a trauma which contributes to the whole of the individual.

These layers are not static structures, however. They are best thought of as vibrational *wheels within wheels*. As such they are in constant motion, still exerting some effect since they are in a constant state of 'oneness' with the whole self. Because of the different defence mechanisms in operation, their effect may have been almost nullified, yet the potential is always there for it to be released.

Imagine several emotions are being held in the unconscious, each of them vibrating on its own but contributing to the overall vibrational pattern. A new emotional assault, trauma or event occurs which produces a sudden alteration in the overall vibrational pattern. As a result, there is a weakening of the defences and one of the vibrational layers is released, or 'fragments' to allow 'bubbles' of emotion to break through into the consciousness. This may be associated with an effect upon the physical body and the manifestation of a physical problem which may have been associated with that buried emotion. This in turn may alter the vibrational pattern of other layers to cause other symptoms to appear.

We return, therefore, to the concept of *maya* which we discussed in Chapter 3. Existence as we know it is an illusion. The underlying reality is that the individual is a composite of all his past physical and emotional experiences. These things do not disappear, but they affect our continued development throughout life.

Strategies in homoeopathy – what to treat

In the homoeopathic treatment of emotional problems we have two main approaches. Firstly, we can use the constitutional remedy to 'set the ball rolling.' Alternatively, (if the constitutional remedy is not obvious) we can treat the predominant emotion (be that jealousy, guilt, hate, etc) or the outward manifestation of that emotional problem.

Both approaches are valid, but it is important to appreciate that there may be different outcomes. With the constitutional remedy, for example, since it accords with the individual's overall profile and works at the very heart and soul of the problem, there may well be temporary flare-ups of past burned-out problems. An old skin eruption might break out, for example.

Treating the predominant emotion or the outward symptoms of the problem is likely to soften the problem in the short-term. That is, it is quite likely to reappear again after some time, unless a second remedy is given to deal with the 'onion layer' immediately below. Think of this approach as being akin to peeling away the layers of the onion.

This model of treatment can be seen in Figure 2.

Of course, if the wrong remedy is chosen then nothing will

Fig. 2

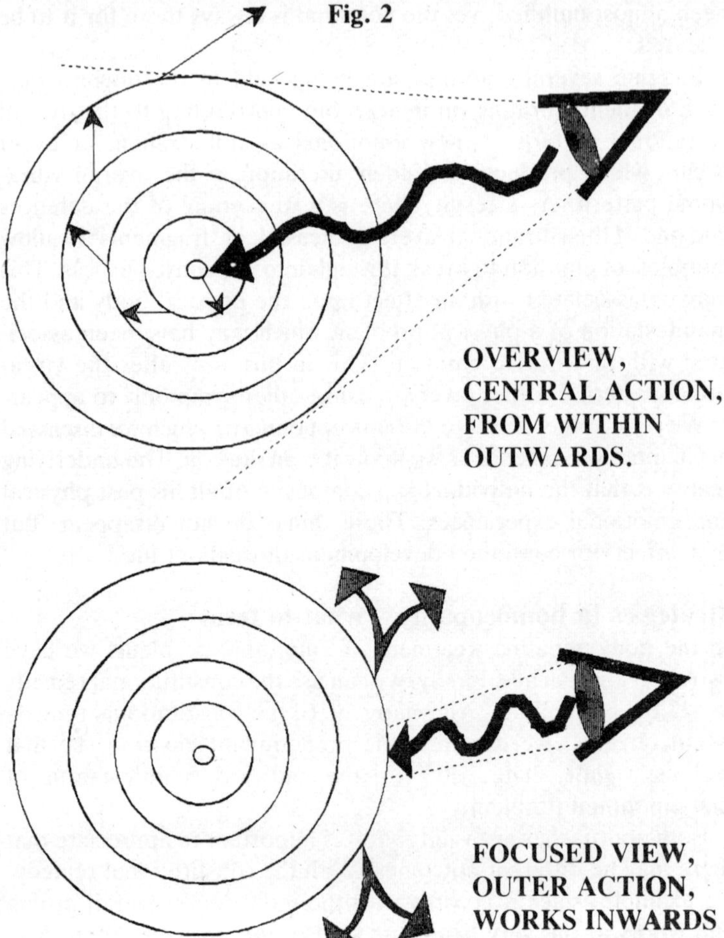

happen. The message is simple. Try as hard as you can to get the exact remedy, the similimum. If this happens to be the constitutional remedy then the chances of ultimate cure are excellent. If it is more a 'pathological' remedy, then success will follow if the match is good. However, one should be ready for the release of other emotions once redundant psychological defense mechanisms 'release their load.'

Coping With Stress

Stress is often talked about these days. People are aware that this thing called stress can damage their health. They are also conscious of the fact that some people seem to 'cope' better with it than others. Well, it is true, some types of people can ride any stressful situation while others seem to flounder at the first stage. It may be, however, that the two types may be closer than one thinks in terms of actual ability to withstand stress, it is just that one person has better 'coping mechanisms' than the other.

There is an important point to understand here. Simply, it is the fact that *stress*, which can be physical, psychological, emotional or spiritual, produces problems when it produces *strain*. Let us use another model to demonstrate this.

Imagine that stress is a force which can move a ball from point A to its resting place at point B. Assume that the farther the ball travels the greater will be the strain felt by the individual. If that ball travels in a completely straight path, then clearly it will travel the greatest distance to produce the most strain. (Fig. 3a)

This situation represents the vulnerable individual who has no defence against stress.

If, however, the individual has a coping mechanism, some means of diverting the path of the ball so that it has to travel to point C before reaching B, then the ultimate distance between A and B will be much shorter. (Fig. 3b) More than that, if he has extra coping mechanisms which cause the ball to have to travel through points D and E as well, then the ultimate strain felt because of the shortened distance between A and B will be much less. (Fig. 3c)

As stated earlier, some people are more resilient. It may be that their psychological defence mechanisms are more effective, or they have other coping mechanisms which buffer stress to minimise the strain they feel. Both are more fortunate than those devoid of the ability to cope.

But most people do find some sort of coping mechanism. Giving oneself adequate breaks in the working day is one method, as is talking to a friend, playing squash, golf or going for a swim. If the coping mechanism is some sort of interest, then it helps to disconnect from the stresses which produce strain in the daily life. These sort of things are all good, potentially strong coping mechanisms.

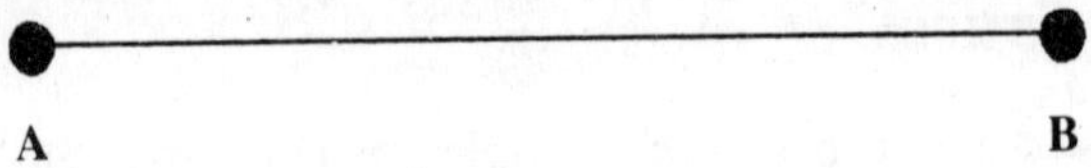

Fig. 3a

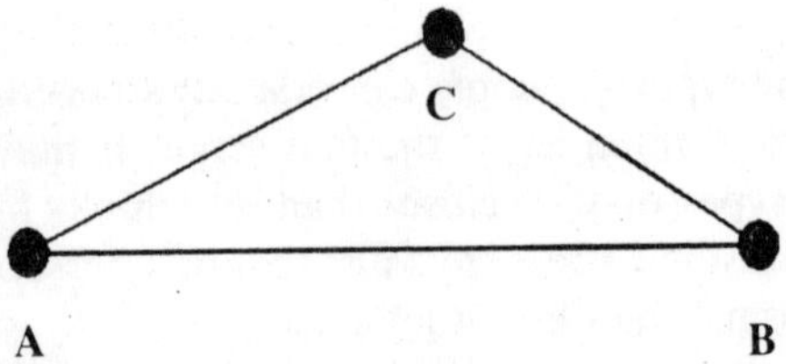

Fig 3b

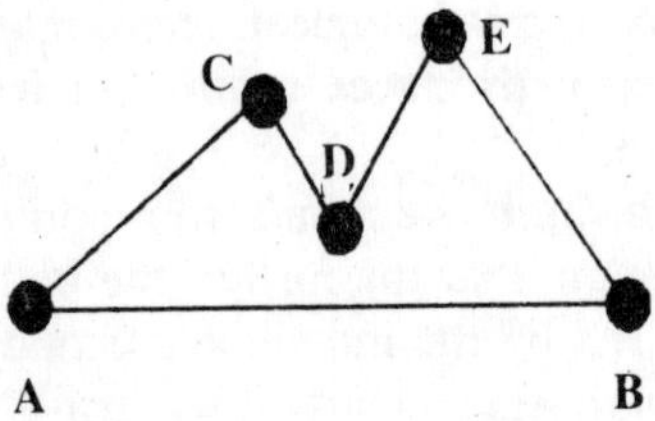

Fig 3c

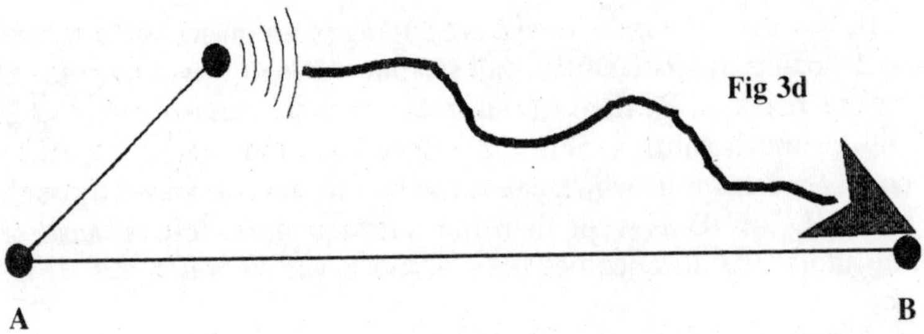

Fig 3d

Clearly, from what we discussed earlier, physically active coping mechanisms lean heavily upon the defense mechanism of sublimation.

On the other hand, some people may adopt things which help them to cope in the short term, but which ultimately produce further strain of their own accord. Here we have the addictions to coffee, tobacco, alcohol and harder drugs. While they can ease the physical and psychological strain in the immediate period, they cause their own strain as physical and psychological dependency develop. There then follows a need to have a regular 'fix,' followed by a shortening of the time between doses and the inevitable escalation. If the regular dose is missed, then a withdrawal effect follows with its unpleasant feelings. It does not then take long before one is a slave to the drug – whichever one it happens to be.

Thus, while a habit initially acts as a good coping mechanism (Fig 3b), it will eventually become a stress in itself which will produce its own strain. Indeed, the net effect will be to heighten the overall strain felt by the individual (Fig 3d).

It is important to try to cultivate good coping mechanisms to offset the effect of stress. In my opinion, however, it is not possible to lay down a blueprint for the best coping mechanisms, because different constitutional types have different preferences and different needs. From the last chapter you may have noted that Arsenicum album types are very neat and fastidious. An activity which was at variance with that would probably only heighten their stress, so they may not enjoy some of the 'messier' outdoor activities. Yoga might be suitable for them. On the other hand, Sepia types tend to become withdrawn and introspective, so that yoga could be a poor coping mechanism, whereas a dance class would probably suit them exactly.

In choosing good coping mechanisms one almost needs to heed the advice of the Delphic Oracle – *Know thyself*.

Protective emotions

It is also a fact that some emotions spring to the fore in order to protect the individual. The obvious example here is anxiety. Often when someone becomes depressed they sink so low that it can become quite dangerous for them to become too inward looking. Their self esteem can reach rock bottom and they could end up wondering whether it is worth going on with life. The mind, finding this to be threatening, freezes the tendency to look inwards by developing a protective shell of anxiety. Thus, like a spiky, barbed wire barrier it stops the individual from examining themselves too much. As long as they don't look inwards they may feel reasonable, but if they let themselves go, they will feel the panic which forces them to focus their minds elsewhere.

Indeed, this is one of the dangers of tranquillisers, because they reduce the protective outer shell of anxiety which allows the individual to look inwards without the fear. Since the depression can then be looked at 'in cold blood,' so to speak, they may then think that there is a reason for feeling such lack of self-esteem. The result could be the impulse to harm oneself.

Yet another example is the effect of the destructive emotion of guilt. Very often it proves to be such a devastating emotion that a protective shell of anger surrounds it. The result is that the individual becomes embittered, irritable and quite impossible to live with.

The causes of emotions

So far I have mentioned little about the causes of emotions. I have not talked about primal injuries, oedipal complexes, substitute gratification, sexual abuse, and the legion of other things which could cause a person to suffer from an emotional problem. The reason is that while these are obviously important, the crucial thing in homoeopathy is the *reaction* of the individual. While the defence mechanisms are important, the main thing we look at is the overall perception of life. Effectively, we are looking at the facade, the front that is projected to the world, and at the 'feelings' which the individual has about themselves, the world and their interaction with it. Thus, we are trying to get at the heart and soul of the problem. When you can do that and match up the appropriate remedy-profile, you are likely to have the *similar*.

That is the whole aim of homoeopathy.

PART TWO

SPECIFIC EMOTIONAL PROBLEMS

CHAPTER 6

Fear

> *"Let me assert my firm belief that the only thing we have to fear is fear itself."*
>
> Franklin D. Roosevelt,
> *US Presidential Address, 1933*

Fear is a universal emotion. Every human being will have experienced it at some stage in their life. The person who has never known fear is a fictional character. Indeed, the concept of bravery exists because it necessitates some act in a situation which most people would consider to be dangerous or fear-inducing.

In Chapter 1 we looked at fear in terms of its psychological, physiological and behavioural components. To recap, when exposed to a certain situation or thought, the individual begins to experience the feeling that something unpleasant is about to happen. This induces the desire to either remove oneself from the situation, or alter the situation in order to reduce the feeling of impending unpleasantness.

Physiologically, the adrenal glands start releasing adrenaline into the circulation. This stimulates the *sympathetic nervous system* which speeds up the heart, quickens the breathing and enhances the eyesight by dilating the pupils. At the same time it inhibits the *parasympathetic nervous system*, thereby reducing the production of saliva and other 'vegetative' functions of the body. Thus, the body is prepared physically for *fight or flight*.

Finally, the psychological and physiological components, the feeling and the sensation of fear, allow the individual to make the choice as to whether to face up to the situation or to 'run for it.'

The actual response makes up the behavioural component.

This is of course a very simplistic analysis of fear. Although everyone will have experienced something akin to this, the way that they actually feel it is unique to them. People have different thresholds for fear, different susceptibilities in differing situations and a tendency to use different unconscious defence mechanisms. In addition, people utilise the coping mechanisms that they find work best for them. (See Chapters 4 and 5.)

The many faces of fear

The word anxiety is derived from the latin *anxietas*, meaning troubled in mind. This in turn seems to have been derived from Sanskrit and Greek roots. As an emotion it was well described by Hippocrates who felt that while it was a type of fear, it was not the same as the state of panic or terror.

Indeed, there seems to be more to it than a matter of degree. Like love, fear seems to have many forms.

Psychiatrists differentiate between normal fear, and abnormal or pathological fear.

Normal fear is construed as the appropriate temporary emotion which people feel when exposed to certain situations or circumstances which they perceive to be in some way threatening. Many people are in fact able to use this usefully to their advantage. For example, actors and sportsmen can 'psyche themselves up' prior to an event, so that they use the circulating adrenaline to actually enhance their performance capability. Essentially, their coping mechanisms are so appropriately tuned in those particular circumstances that they suffer no ill effects and actually 'enjoy' their emotion.

Abnormal fear, by contrast, is viewed as the experience of fear either in an inappropriate situation, or out of proportion to the situation.

In general, at least 75 per cent of people consulting their doctor have anxiety to some degree. Of that figure the majority will be experiencing 'normal' fear in association with their perception of illness. A significant proportion, however, some 10–15 per cent will be suffering from abnormal fear at a level to be construed as an illness in itself. Most studies on the female:male ratio show that females consult more frequently with such abnormal fear problems in the proportion of 3.5:1.

In recent years it has been assumed that anxiety and abnormal fear is a product of modern living. It was assumed that the stresses of living in a developed, so-called 'advanced' culture caused burn-out, break-downs and panic states in unprecedented numbers. It was suggested that since modern stressful situations are less physically dangerous than in the days when lions and tigers had to be encountered, we began suppressing the physiological component of our fear emotion. In other words, since there were few situations in the concrete jungle when one had to fight or actually flee, the psychological component took on the added load to produce a more exaggerated perception of the emotion of fear. The theory developed that the 'concrete jungle' had created more stress-related illness than the halcyon days of our ancestors.

When epidemiologists started looking at this, however, it was shown to be untrue. Abnormal fear states have always been with us. Indeed, in comparing developed with developing countries the overall prevalence is much the same. Between 15 and 20 per cent of people suffer from it to such a degree that they seek aid.

Undoubtedly, this figure is still only the tip of the iceberg. Many people feel excessive fear, but would never dream of contacting a doctor because they do not consider it to be abnormal for them. The fact is, however, that it may be abnormal, but since they have always lived with it they have developed coping mechanisms to minimise it. This may mean that they avoid relationships, situations and opportunities and end up leading a less than satisfied life because they 'fear the fear' which they 'know' would follow.

As we shall see later, among other ways fear may manifest itself as a generalised anxiety state, as a phobia, as a tendency to suffer from panic attacks, or as an illness fear.

Breathing – a natural coping mechanism

In Chapter 5, I mentioned that coping mechanisms are most effective when they are in tune with the needs of the individual's constitutional type. I cited the example of yoga being perhaps an inappropriate activity for some people. I stand by this, because I simply do not believe that there are many activities which would benefit 'everyone.' Having said that, I think that *yogic breathing* could help *most* people control or minimise their fear.

Yoga is a collection of physical, contemplative and meditative techniques, the origins of which at least date back some 5,000 years. There are 8 'limbs' or branches of yoga, one of which is called *pranayama* – the science of breath control.

Essentially, pranayama teaches one to control one's breathing. It is an excellent thing to try to do, since controlled breathing can alleviate the ravages of stress and modify the individual's reaction to it in order to minimise strain.

To begin with, one should note the emphasis upon the word 'control' since it means more than the unconscious process of inhaling and exhaling.

Basically, there are two forms of breathing – *thoracic*, where the ribcage actually expands and contracts; and *diaphragmatic*, where the ribcage is more or less motionless while the abdomen expands and contracts.

Chest-breathers seem to breathe at an average rate of 12–16 full breaths a minute, whereas diaphragmatic-breathers only need about 8–10 breaths a minute. If you add that up, there is a significant 'saving of breath' and energy for the diaphragmatic-breathers.

Try the following simple exercise and I think you will be surprised at how relaxed you can make yourself.

Firstly, sit in a comfortable chair somewhere away from noise. Place the hands flat on the abdomen just below the navel, with the fingertips touching.

Now inhale slowly through the nose, at the same time pushing the abdomen out so that the fingertips separate. Make sure that you keep your back straight, since this will help the lungs fill with air, and continue to expand the chest and abdomen even after you think you have inhaled deeply.

Now raise the shoulders and hold the breath for five seconds. Then slowly exhale through the nose and begin to draw in the abdomen.

Let all the air empty out by exhaling more deeply than usual and, when you think it has all gone, hold your breath for a second or two before you inhale again.

If you learn to control your breathing, by doing these exercises for about five minutes twice a day, your breathing pattern will begin to change, you will generally feel more relaxed and you will have developed a simple coping mechanism.

PANIC

Sudden, acute fear can be difficult to deal with. If it occurs following an acute physical or mental trauma, then it is likely to be quite short-lived. On the other hand, about 5 per cent of the population regularly suffer from sudden acute attacks of panic which hit them out of the blue.

The psychological and physical components of an acute panic attack are very marked. There is sudden, overwhelming dread and terror. Accompanying it there is a virtual explosion of sympathetic nerve stimulation. Thus, the individual might experience some or all of the following symptoms and signs:- dizziness, palpitations, perspiration, trembling, pallor, the urge to vomit, open the bowels or pass water.

In addition, there may be tingling and pins and needles felt in the limbs and around the mouth. This is generally caused by over-breathing as the individual gasps for air. Effectively, this causes the lungs to blow off all the carbon dioxide (CO_2) reserve. When this happens, a state of *alkalosis* is brought about, wherein the blood becomes slightly alkaline. In turn, this affects the chemistry of calcium within the blood-stream, resulting in a process which causes hyper-excitability of the nerves. This causes the sensation of tingling and an unpleasant cramp in the hands and face. At its worst, the hands become temporarily drawn into a claw-shape. Unfortunately, because this is so alarming, it may cause the individual's panic to intensify.

Panic attacks are usually self-limiting in a few minutes as the body's internal regulatory mechanisms begin to restore the acid-base balance and the blood chemistry to normal. Some people, however, may experience their attacks for several hours.

One of the best ways of dealing with a panic attack is controlled breathing. Initially, breathing in and out into one's own cupped hands is advisable, since this will tend to concentrate the CO_2, so that the reserve is not lost.

If someone is subject to repeated attacks, then I would certainly advocate learning a good breathing technique such as the one I described above.

The four following remedies are particularly useful. As in all homoeopathic prescribing, however, it is important to pay particular attention to the reaction of the individual. Quite simply, if the remedy-profile doesn't match the patient-profile it will not work.

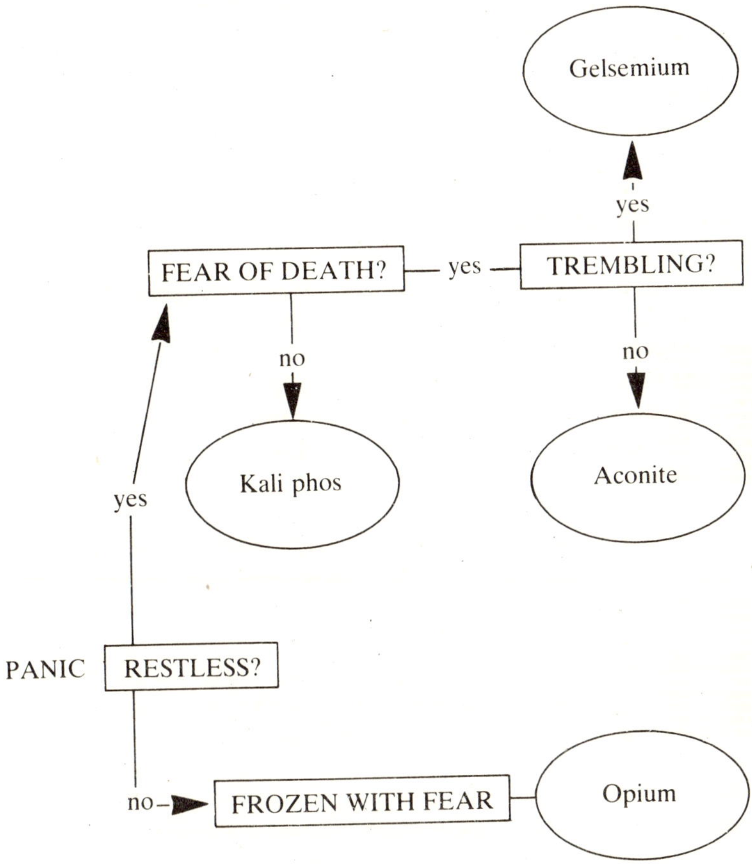

PANIC

Aconite – for the fear accompanying a sudden shock. There is restlessness, palpitations and a fear of death. A fever may develop with the fear. An excellent remedy for agitated panic attacks. Also very useful for those who wake in a cold sweat, with their blankets in disarray after a nightmare.

Gelsemium – for panic attacks which render the individual exhausted. They will feel themselves to be 'trembling with fear.'

Kali phosphoricum – for panic attacks in very nervous types, subject to night terrors. May become hysterical.

Opium – for panic where the individual is 'petrified with fear,' 'rooted to the spot,' or 'frozen with terror'.

Fear in Anticipation

Many people are able to take events and engagements in their stride. Others might never give the event a moments thought until the event is actually upon them. Still others might dwell upon the event for days or even weeks ahead, their anxiety level mounting all the time, or becoming more intense every time they think about it. These people might well benefit from one of the following remedies:-

Argentum nitricum – for anxiety days before an event, causing diarrhoea. There may also be palpitations and increased perspiration.

Gelsemium – for anxiety days before an event, causing the need to pass urine frequently. Will tremble with anxiety whenever the event is contemplated. Sleep will probably suffer.

Kali phosphoricum – for anxiety and dread days before events, especially if having to meet people for the first time. Can become very lethargic. May suffer night terrors.

Lycopodium – for anxiety days before in reserved, worried looking professional types (eg, teachers, solicitors, doctors). Often very conscientious and sensitive. Even although they may be used to public speaking, etc, they will still be subject to the anticipatory anxiety. Once they start the event, however, they will perform perfectly well. May be prone to stomach ulcers and digestive complaints.

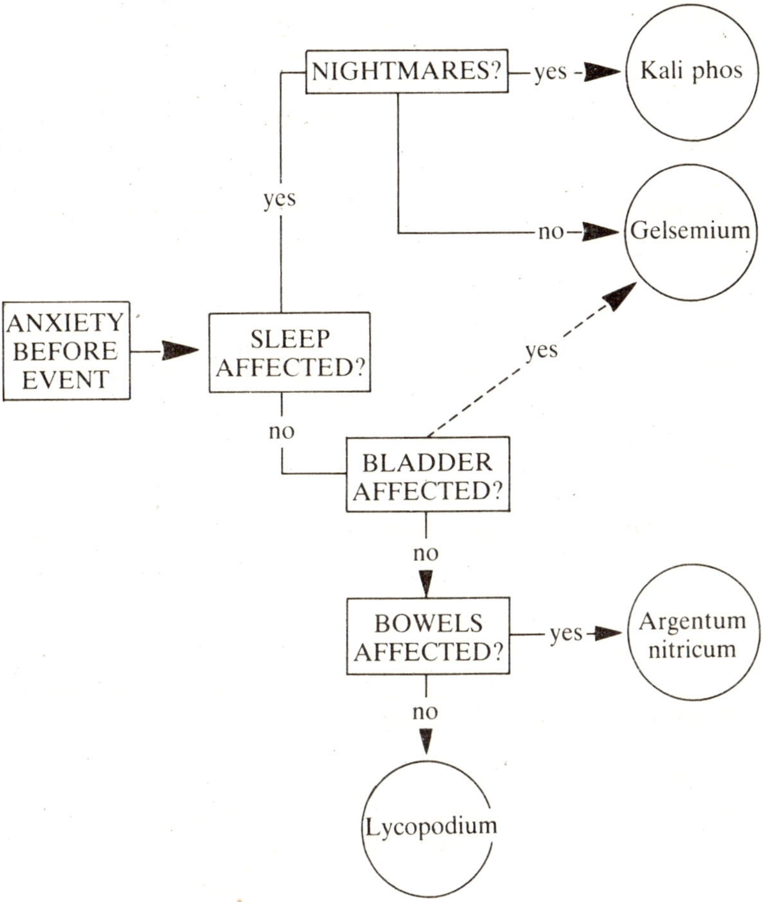

ANTICIPATORY FEAR

BOTTLED-UP ANXIETY

It is an old axiom of folk medicine that one should never 'bottle up' an emotion. Fear, it is said, can burn into you to produce all sorts of problems. Indeed, some people bottle-up their emotions so successfully that an emotional problem may only come to light after a secondary medical complication has occurred.

Causticum – for generalised anxiety states in shy, pessimistic types. They are often weepy. They are always extremely sympathetic about other people. Thinking about their own ailments, however, always makes them worse – especially warts and haemorrhoids.

Gelsemium – for generalised anxiety states in listless, trembly types. They may have to lie down when stressed. Strong emotions will make them feel ill, particularly making them prone to 'flu', migraine and diarrhoea.

Lycopodium – for generalised anxiety states in reserved, worried looking professional types (eg, teachers, solicitors, doctors). Often very conscientious and sensitive. May be prone to stomach ulcers and digestive complaints.

Natrum muriaticum – for generalised anxiety states in touchy, melancholic types. They dislike sympathy, which always makes them feel worse. They may want to be alone to cry. They crave salt and salty foods. They may be prone to migraine and typically 'hammering headaches,' skin problems and depression.

Phosphorus – for generalised anxiety states in sensitive, creative or artistic types. They dread death and hate being alone. Their sensitivity may manifest itself by reacting to loud noises, storms or arguments. May have sudden flare-ups of temper, which disappear just as quickly as they come. They may be prone to nose-bleeds, period problems, laryngitis.

Pulsatilla – for generalised anxiety states in gentle, yielding types. They weep easily at sad films, music and upon reading about tragedies in the newspapers. They are generally better for sympathy. They may be prone to anaemia, catarrh and styes.

Restless Anxiety

While the above remedies are suitable for those people who try to put on a brave face, the following are more appropriate when the reaction is one of restlessness or agitation.

Arsenicum album – for generalised anxiety states when there is marked restlessness in a tidy, fussy type. They tend to despair, particularly about their health and feel that not enough is being done to help.

Bryonia – for generalised anxiety states where the individual cannot keep still, despite the fact that movement may make their symptoms worse. They may be quite irritable, but anger will make them worse.

Calcarea carbonica – for generalised anxiety states where the individual feels sensitive about people looking at them. They may wring their hands as they think or talk about their anxieties. They may fear that they are going mad. They generally feel worse in the evening and are worse for exertion, either physical or mental.

Iodum – for generalised anxiety states where the individual feels worse for inactivity. They have to keep busy and may feel compelled to act on impulse. They may even become aggressive on impulse.

Sexual Fears

Relationship difficulties are a frequent cause of emotional problems. On the other hand, emotional problems can often cause difficulties within relationships. In this area sexual fears can be particularly devastating.

It should be appreciated, however, that the sexual fear may in itself merely be a sign of another emotional problem, such as depression. If this is the case, then that problem should be the target of treatment in the first instance.

Male problems

There are two main difficulties experienced by men. Firstly, there is *premature ejaculation*, in which the man ejaculates before or immediately upon penetration. Secondly, there is *erectile impotence*, in which there is an inability to obtain or maintain an erection.

Both may be the result of anticipatory or performance fear. A

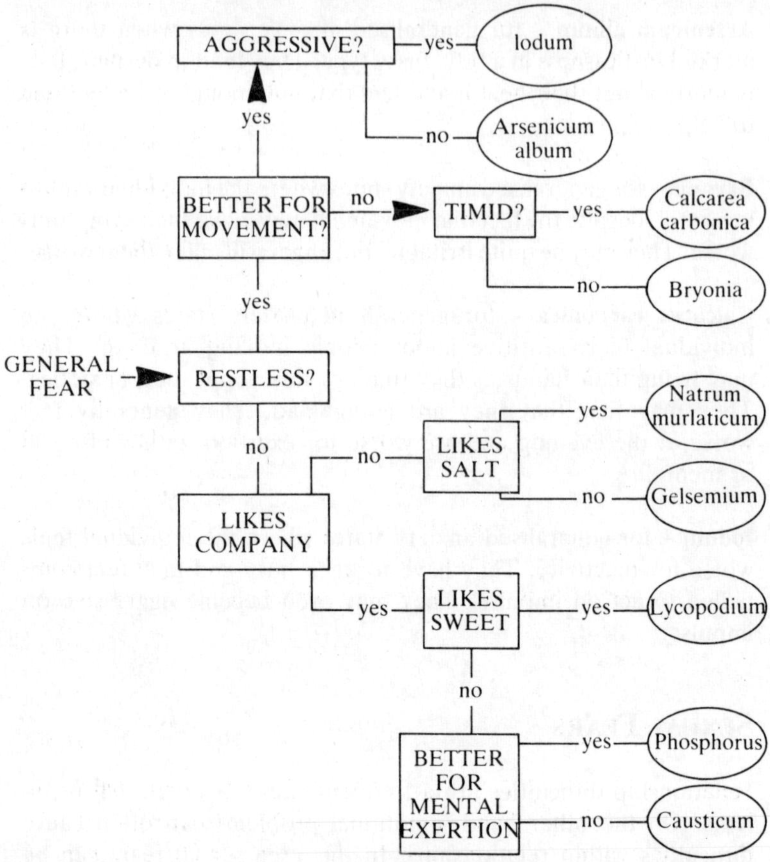

GENERALISED ANXIETY

vicious circle may thereby be set up, because each time the problem occurs there will be a 'fear load' which will further reduce the chances of overcoming the difficulty.

About 75 per cent of males ejaculate within two minutes of sexual penetration. The aim of treatment in premature ejaculation is to increase the length of time that the erection can be maintained.

A useful thing to do is for the couple to mutually agree not to actually have intercourse. Foreplay is to be encouraged, with the intention of obtaining an erection but with only just enough stimulation so that an orgasm is not achieved. Stimulation is then withdrawn so that the erection starts to recede. Over time, these foreplay sessions are increased until such mild stimulation results in an erection being maintained for up to about twenty minutes at a time. Only then should actual intercourse be contemplated.

There are various drugs which can cause erectile impotence. For example, some antidepressants, steroids and antihypertensives.

UNDER NO CIRCUMSTANCES, HOWEVER, SHOULD MEDICATION BE STOPPED WITHOUT CONSULTING YOUR DOCTOR.

In addition to this, certain medical problems need to be excluded, including – alcohol dependence, diabetes mellitis, vascular diseases, neurological disease and various endocrine problems.

IF THERE IS A COMPLAINT OF ERECTILE IMPOTENCE, THEN A MEDICAL OPINION SHOULD BE SOUGHT.

The following homoeopathic remedies might help.

Argentum nitricum – for sexual problems in one who experiences much anticipatory fear. There may be palpitations at the thought of sex, possibly also with the feeling of queeziness in the abdomen.

Lycopodium – for both erectile impotence (usually merely a weak erection) and premature ejaculation in worried, intellectual types. They may become jealous of other 'less able' people who clearly have no such problems. They may tend to be quite haughty.

Phosphoric acidum – for sexual fear in lethargic, indifferent types. A shock or grief may have caused the problem.

Female problems

The main problem here is *vaginismus*, in which the pelvic muscles contract to the extent that sexual intercourse is impossible.

Gynaecological problems, perhaps causing *dyspareunia*, pain on intercourse, have to be considered. In addition, past psychological traumas, including sexual abuse, may be the cause.

A medical opinion should always be the starting point.

I have found that the following two remedies can be of use.

Belladonna – for acute vaginismus, with blushing, hotness and acute fear. It may come on suddenly without any evidence of anticipatory fear.

Cactus grandiflorus – for vaginismus in melancholic types. The vaginismus is severe and may be quite painful, as if the muscles have gone into a constricting spasm. May even scream out in pain.

CHAPTER 7

Phobias

Men fear Death, as children fear to go in the dark; and as that natural fear in children is increased with tales, so is the other.

Sir Francis Bacon, *Of Death*

A phobia is defined as the experience of persistent excessive fear when in contact with an object or situation which is not in itself a significant source of danger.

As mentioned in Chapter 1, the name is derived from the Ancient Greek deity *Phobos*, a son of Ares, the god of war. It was believed that he was responsible for striking soldiers with abject terror. There was, however, a difference between the fear he was associated with, and that caused by the other deity, *Pan*. While Pan could cause 'panic attacks' without warning under virtually any circumstance, Phobos only caused fear in a particular situation.

This is quite an important distinction to make, since the two problems are often confused. Although the fear that is felt can be exactly the same, phobias always have a recognisable and repeated trigger, whereas the panic attack comes out of the blue (See Chapter 6).

Like all types of fear, phobias can be looked at in terms of the three components mentioned in Chapters 1 and 6, ie, the psychological *feeling*, the physiological *sensation* and the behavioural *action*. The characteristic thing about phobias, however, is that because the individual knows how they will feel if exposed to a particular situation they are able to take the appropriate action to avoid it. Indeed, people with phobias may never actually feel fear, because they completely avoid the situations which are liable to trigger the fear reaction. In other words they structure their whole life to live around their fear, rather than risk facing up to it. Further than that, they may be so successful at avoiding their problem that friends and relatives may not even be aware that there is a problem.

It has to be said that unless the individual admits that there is a problem, there is little likelihood of it disappearing! So that is step one – admit that there is a phobia and accept the help of other people in helping to deal with it.

Sometimes phobias occur on their own and sometimes they occur as a symptom of another emotional problem. For example, depression can often be accompanied by the development of a phobia. This is an example of one of the mixed emotions I alluded to in Chapter 5. In this case the phobia makes one avoid a particular situation which might make the depression worse. Thus, the phobic symptom acts as a protective element. As we shall see later, this has significance in the way one should approach treatment.

Types of phobia

Generally, it is accepted that there are three main types of phobic fear.

1) Agoraphobia and claustrophobia
2) Specific phobias
3) Social phobias

There is yet another group of conditions which could be categorised as a 'miscellaneous group', but I feel that they are more to do with an obsessive-compulsive sort of problem, so they shall be the subject of the next chapter on Fixations.

Treatment of phobias

There are many treatments advocated for phobic fear. Psychotherapy may help by getting to the root of the problem, but it tends to be time-consuming and may be quite traumatic as inner problems are exposed and analysed. Hypnosis can also be used, but is most effective for simple or single phobias. Only trained therapists should attempt such treatment.

Behavioural treatment is the method used by most psychologists, who usually arrange some form of graded exposure. This is a step-by-step approach whereby the sufferer gradually works through a program until they finally feel able to expose themselves fully to the feared situation.

A behavioural approach is in fact my preferred style of management, combined with homoeopathy. And this is where it is as well to have friends or relatives involved. It is important, however, that they understand that the phobic sufferer cannot simply be told to get on with it. The nature of a phobia is that it is very difficult to be logical and rational about the feared situation. Even although the sufferer knows that nothing bad can really happen logically, they cannot bring themselves to believe that this is the case. A genuine, understanding helper is therefore worth their weight in gold.

Together the sufferer and helper should work out a strategy of help. This means in the beginning getting the sufferer to imagine the feared situation. Just that. Merely picture the situation in the mind's eye and tell yourself that nothing bad can happen. While picturing this try the breathing exercises outlined in Chapter 6, and actively let yourself go. Try to relax.

The next step is to try to get photographs of the dreaded place, situation or activity. Look at the pictures in books from the library. Touch the photographs and imagine being there.

Then slowly, over time work out your graded program. At first it should be a matter of going to look at the place, situation or activity from a distance, accompanied by a friend. Then again over time, when you are ready, go nearer, then walk away. Next time go further. Then go there with the friend, walk past or touch the feared thing or do the activity – all the time being aware that the friend is there as well, so the situation is controlled.

Ultimately, with the friend nearby the situation may be attempted – and conquered.

Homoeopathy has a big part to play, simply in restoring balance so that the fear doesn't become disabling. Indeed, if the remedy is well-matched, the problem may simply melt away.

The ideal remedy is the constitutional remedy, since this will work at the heart of the problem. However, if it is not possible to select this, then one can choose the remedy which most closely matches the pattern of the phobia. In this case one is approaching the problem from the outside of the 'layer model' (see Chapter 5), so one has to be aware that as the phobia disappears, a deeper emotion may seem to come to the surface. This may make the selection of the constitutional remedy clearer. If not, then one can again approach the problem by focusing on the next 'layer' which is presented. (See notes about which potency at the start of Part 3.)

1) Agoraphobia

The term agoraphobia was first coined by a German neurologist by the name of Carl Westphal. He derived it from the Greek word *agora*, which meant meeting or marketplace. And that is what it is, a fear of open or public places.

Three-quarters of all sufferers are females. The commonest age affected are those between 25 and 35 years. There is a tendency for it to run in families, so that it is not uncommon to have three generations of women who have been affected

Aconite – for the fear of going out, or going into a public place when there is a feeling of certainty that death or injury will inevitably happen.

Arnica – for the fear of going out because of the memory of some accident or trauma.

Arsenicum album – where there is acute restlessness. They will fuss about the home and get annoyed if anyone tries to get them to go out. Will also be annoyed if people do not fit into their plans.

Lycopodium – where there is a general fear of crowds. On the other hand, they do not like to be left on their own. There is a dislike of having to perform or speak in public. They may agonise for days before an event when they have to go out and may make up any excuse not to have to go.

Natrum muriaticum – where there is a general dislike of company. They tend to be solitary. They hate going anywhere that people might be sympathetic towards them, eg, after a bereavement. Thus, they may just 'pull up the drawbridge' and stay at home.

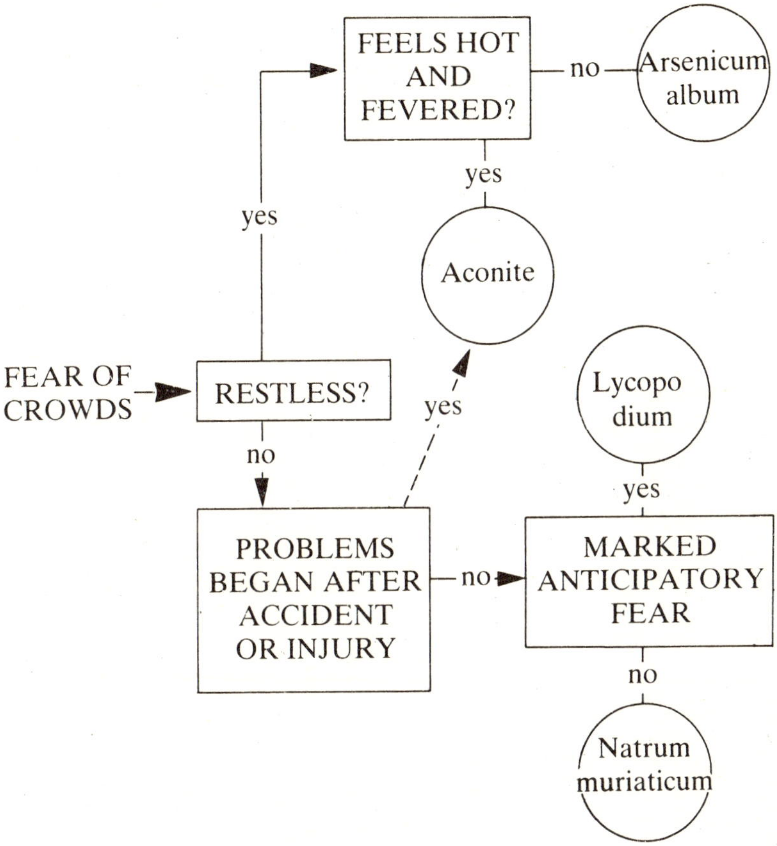

AGORAPHOBIA

CLAUSTROPHOBIA

Claustrophobia means a fear of enclosed spaces. It is derived from the Latin *claustrum*, meaning bolt or lock.

Like agoraphobia it is commoner in females in the age group 25–35 years. It may co-exist with agoraphobia, or alternate with it.

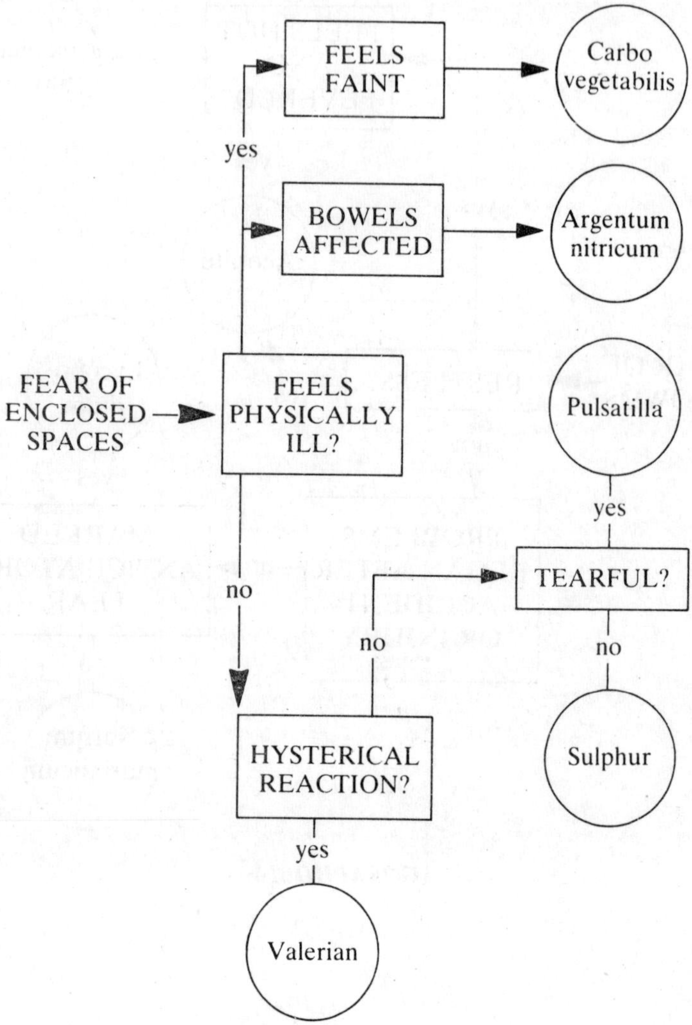

CLAUSTROPHOBIA

Argentum nitricum – for a fear of enclosed spaces when the prospect causes diarrhoea. They will feel the need to rapidly get to fresh air, so that they will want to ensure a ready escape route.

Carbo vegetabilis – for a fear of enclosed spaces when the individual feels as if they may faint or collapse. They may come out in a cold sweat.

Pulsatilla – for a fear of enclosed spaces in a changeable, weepy individual. They hate stuffy environments and are always better outdoors. They are rarely thirsty.

Sulphur – for a fear of enclosed spaces in generally dominant type people. They are expansive and dislike being hemmed in. They find it difficult to be still and will always tend to lean or slouch.

Valerian – for a fear of enclosed spaces in individuals who react hysterically when confronted by the object of their fear.

Specific Phobias

Very specific fears are commonest in young children of both sexes before they reach puberty. They will generally clear up spontaneously, but until they do they can create immense problems for the family. The type of fear they induce is usually terror.

The correct homoeopathic remedy will often work absolute wonders. The constitutional remedy is certainly worth giving if it can be worked out, although this is not always easy in children.

Specific phobias in adults may, in fact, be symptoms of other more deep-rooted anxiety states. If there does seem to be anxiety about other things, then again the constitutional remedy is more appropriate.

The following phobias may respond well to the following remedies.

Animals – (*Zoophobia*)

Shakespeare talks about a fear of cats in his play, The Merchant of Venice. It is a common phobia among children and women of all ages.

Many people have phobias about dogs and of being bitten by them.

Causticum – for general fear of animals in children who hate to go to bed on their own. They are always worse if they think about their illnesses and ailments, so they are better when distracted.

China officinalis – for general fear of animals and all 'creepie-crawlies'. The fear is always worse at night. They are always worse after an illness where they have lost body fluids or blood.

Hyoscyamus – for general fear of animals in children who laugh and giggle a lot. They tend to argue about everything and may mumble to themselves. They may fear being bitten or scratched.

Stramonium – for general fear in children who stammer and always want company. They may fear that they will be eaten by the animals.

Insects and Spiders

Fear of bees and wasps are common, possibly after being stung. There also seems to be an inborn wariness of these creatures which have the yellow and black markings which are nature's 'Warning colours.'

Flies and blue-bottles are the next commonest, especially among the very young.

Moth phobias are far commoner than butterfly phobias, presumably because they are creatures of the night.

Spider phobias are common in childhood, although many adults (women more than men) retain the fear throughout life.

Argentum nitricum – for fear of insects or spiders in people who tend to get diarrhoea when they are frightened. Since they also tend to fear enclosed spaces, they may get extremely upset if confronted by such creatures when they are in a room on their own.

Gelsemium – for fear of insects or spiders in people who will fly into a panic and shake like a leaf. They will need to lie down.

Nux vomica – for fear of insects or spiders in people who tend to be irritable if it is suggested that they are frightened of anything.

Burglars

Arsenicum album – for people who tend to fear that people might have broken in. They tend to sleep with their hands and feet underneath the blankets – just in case!

Lachesis – for talkative types who tend to be suspicious. They tend to feel bloated and can get very cross. They would get furious at the thought of someone breaking in.

Mercurius solubilis – for fear of burglars in slow, weary types. They are generally distrustful of people. They tend to suffer from tremors and discharges from various parts of the body.

Natrum muriaticum – for fear of burglars in melancholic types who are always worse for sympathy. They crave salt.

Phosphorus – for fear of burglars in sensitive, creative types. Their hearing may seem so sensitive to them that they often 'hear' bumps in the night which they immediately perceive to be due to burglars.

Dark

Most children are afraid of the dark. Many 'sensitive' types may retain this fear into adulthood.

Aconite – for fear of the dark triggered off after a fright or shock. There will generally be great restlessness.

Calcarea carbonica – for fear of the dark in someone who is slow, suffers from all sorts of 'congestion' and who is generally melancholic. They tend to think that people are looking at them.

Causticum – for fear of the dark in someone who worries and is sympathetic about others, even when they are ill themselves.

Thinking about their fear will usually make them worse. They do not appreciate horror stories or films, which will make them worse.

Lycopodium – for fear of the dark in someone who is sensitive and highly-strung. They fear events in the future, but generally cope when the time comes. They feel pressured to achieve. Often professional types.

Phosphorus – for fear of the dark in someone who is sensitive and creative.

Pulsatilla – for fear of the dark in weepy, timid types who like company and who are better for consolation and sympathy.

Stramonium – for fear of the dark in talkative types who may be afflicted by a stammer.

Death

In youth most people have a sense of immortality, as if nothing can really happen to them. They feel as if they are observers of the mortality of others. This sense can be shaken when one has an accident, a major illness, an operation, or a bereavement. On the other hand, some people always feel vulnerable and view death with abject horror. Still others fear it because of the pressure they place upon their own lives. They are constantly striving to achieve and feel hurried in all the paths of their lives, as if they have so much to do in so short a time.

There are many remedies which have this fear of death. The following are some of the commonest.

Aconite – for fear of death with any illness, however trivial. The fear of death is present, as is the belief that it is soon to come.

Apis mellifica – for fear of death in people who are prone to moan and complain. They may be very clumsy when ill. They tend to be troubled with jealousy and are complainers. They may cry and shriek.

Argentum nitricum – for fear of death in someone who is impulsive and hurried. They may feel so apprehensive that they get diarrhoea.

Arsenicum album – for fear of death in someone who is extremely fussy, neat and restless. They may feel great despair about any treatment.

Bryonia – for fear of death in someone who is worse for any movement. They are capable of bringing on illness through a bout of anger or strong emotion.

Calcarea carbonica – for fear of death in someone who is slow, suffers from all sorts of 'congestion' and who is generally melancholic. They tend to think that people are looking at them.

Causticum – for fear of death in someone who worries and is sympathetic about others, even when they are ill themselves. Thinking about their own illness makes them worse, so they are often better when left to think about others.

Gelsemium – for fear of death in someone who is prostrated when ill. They may tremble with fear at the thought of death. Sometimes, however, they may feel as if their heart could stop, so they force themselves to keep going when all they really want to do is lie down.

Lycopodium – for fear of death in someone who is sensitive and highly-strung. They fear events in the future, but generally cope when the time comes. They feel pressured to achieve. Often professional types.

Nux vomica – for fear of death in irritable, high achievers who tend to use a lot of stimulants. Their tempers can flare up suddenly.

Phosphorus – for fear of death in artistic, sensitive types who are prone to all sorts of bleeding disorders.

Pulsatilla – for fear of death in weepy, timid types who like company and who are better for consolation and sympathy.

Ghosts

Fear of ghosts is again common in 'sensitive' types of people.

Aconite – for fear of ghosts, especially after a fright or shock.

Arsenicum album – for fear of ghosts in fussy, restless types.

Causticum – for fear of ghosts in someone who is always sympathetic about others. Thinking about their problems always makes them worse. They are liable to be affected by ghost or horror books or films, so should avoid them.

Lycopodium – for fear of ghosts in sensitive, highly strung people. They fear events in the future, but generally cope when the time comes. They feel pressured to achieve. Often professional types.

Phosphorus – for fear of ghosts in someone who is sensitive and creative.

Pulsatilla – for fear of ghosts in weepy, timid types who like company and who are better for consolation and sympathy.

Sulphur – for fear of ghosts in dominant types. They find it difficult to be still and tend to slouch, lean or fidget.

Heights

Argentum nitricum – for those who fear heights because they are impulsive and suspect that they may have a 'lemming' impulse to jump off the edge of a cliff or out of a window.

Pulsatilla – for weepy, timid types who fear heights because they feel sure that they could get dizzy and fall off.

Sulphur – for dominant types who may be embarrassed about their fear of heights. They tend to slouch, lean or fidget.

Thunderstorms

Natrum muriaticum – for fear of thunderstorms in melancholic types who are worse for sympathy. They are best left sheltering under the table!

Phosphorus – for fear of thunderstorms in someone who is sensitive and creative. They detest the noise of the thunder and may become ill during the storm.

Rhododendron – for fear of thunderstorms, particularly the thunder in people who are prone to rheumatic disorders. They may have joint problems which are like 'weather barometers.'

Social Phobias

These problems generally relate to fear in the presence of other people. The individual tends to worry about what those around him will think of him. For example, he may fear that he will be thought boring, incompetent, clumsy, stupid or coarse. Sometimes a vicious circle will be created by virtue of the overactivity of the physical component of fear, such as blushing, stammering, having to rush to the toilet, or having to excuse oneself to go and be sick.

Social phobias tend to occur in adults and may be isolated phobias, or symptoms of more general anxiety or depressive states.

Fear of Strangers

Baryta carbonica – for fear of strangers in children and the elderly. Children may seem slow and reserved, while the elderly may seem to have poor memories and poor concentration.

Carbo vegetabilis – for fear of strangers in those who are exhausted. They feel intense fear and may need to fan themselves to 'cool their fear.'

Causticum – for fear of strangers in someone who is always sympathetic about others. Thinking about their problems always makes them worse. They need to be distracted before going out and meeting new people.

Cuprum metallicum – for fear of strangers in someone who is generally morose. They tend to suffer from spasms and constricting pains and often have a metallic, coppery taste in the mouth.

Thuja – for fear of strangers in those who are subject to strange 'fixed' ideas, eg, that they feel as if there is someone or something inside them. They commonly suffer from warts.

Fear of Performing

In this context 'performing' means doing anything under the eyes of other people. This can vary from public speaking or playing sport, to going to the theatre or a restaurant.

Argentum nitricum – for a fear of 'performing' when the prospect causes diarrhoea. They will feel the need to rapidly get to fresh air, so that they will want to ensure a ready escape route. Thus in a theatre they will always want an aisle seat, or a table near a door in a restaurant.

Causticum – for fear of 'performing' in someone who is always sympathetic about others. Thinking about their problems always makes them worse. They need to be distracted before the event or meeting.

Gelsemium – for fear of 'performing' in people who shake like a leaf before the event. They may even have to lie down. Often they will have to pass urine, which may be a large amount.

Lycopodium – for fear of 'performing' in sensitive, highly-strung individuals. They may dread the event for days ahead, but are able to cope when the time comes. They often put themselves into situations and then wonder 'why they do it!'

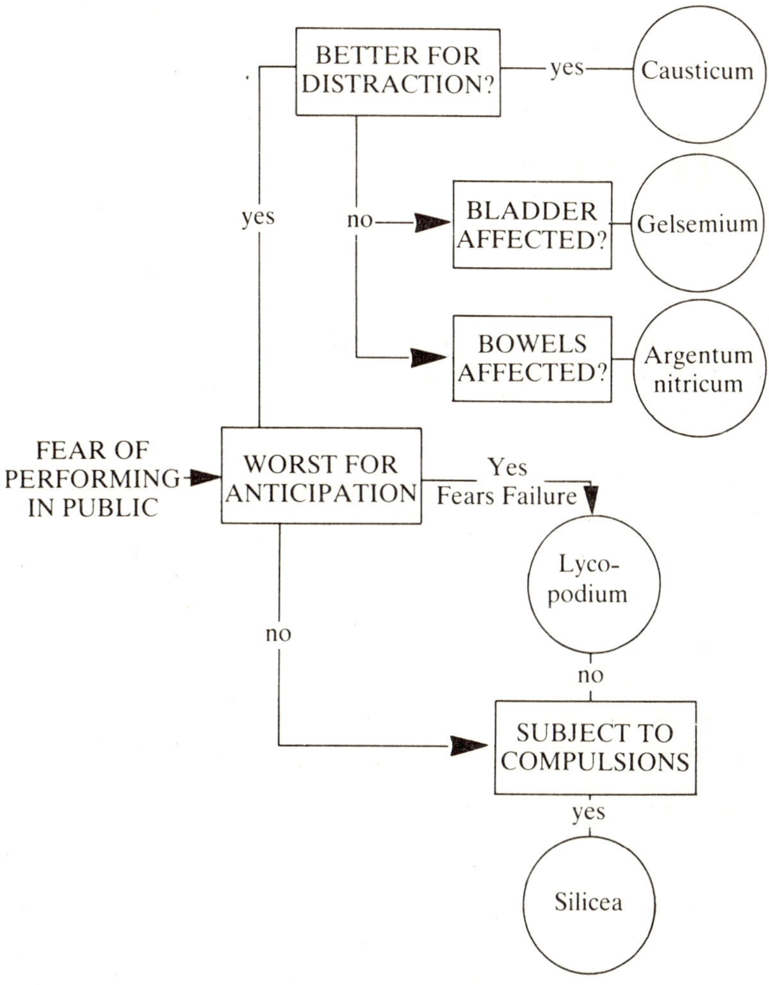

PERFORMING FEAR

Silicea – for fear of 'performing' in sensitive individuals who are always easily discouraged in activities. They may try taking alcohol for 'Dutch courage,' but find that they react badly to it.

CHAPTER 8

Fixations

Out, damned spot! out, I say! One; two: why then, 'tis time to do't. Hell is murky! Fie, my lord, fie! a soldier, and afeard? What need we fear who knows it, when none can call power to account? Yet who would have thought the old man to have had so much blood in him?

William Shakespeare,
Lady Macbeth, Macbeth

William Shakespeare, England's greatest playwright, was undoubtedly one of the greatest observers of mankind. In his plays he describes by word and deed many of the emotional disorders which can afflict we frail human beings. In the play Macbeth, for example, he deals with jealousy and the lust for power, the guilt of the murderer, the fear of ghosts and the gradual deterioration of the mind into the state of madness. Yet although Macbeth's emotional progression is fascinating, the portrayal of Lady Macbeth's obsessive-compulsive behaviour is genius itself. Her delusions, hallucinations and repeated hand-washing could fit well into any contemporary textbook of psychiatry.

Fixations

The term 'fixation' means different things to different people. In Freudian analytical terms it implies an arrest at some point of psychosexual development. In the context of this book, I use it to refer to fixed ideas or impulses which the individual finds difficult to deal with or clear away.

Fixed ideas are commonest in people of tidy, ordered, fussy dispositions. The problem is that they may take over an individual's life to the extent that they are no longer able to function effectively in their jobs, their homes or their relationships.

Many children play the game of avoiding the cracks between paving stones. Similarly, building up a pre-bedtime ritual is common. Both are normal parts of growing up and usually disappear, because they are only ever considered a game. Sometimes, however, they become so strong that they begin to impinge upon the other members of the family, in that if the ritual behaviour is not done quite correctly, the child feels compelled to keep repeating it until it is done to perfection. This is when the obsessive-compulsive behaviour has become fixed as an emotional problem.

Adolescence and early adulthood are also common times for such behaviour to rear its head. Here the obsessive component is usually a fixed thought which may be associated with some superstitious or mystical belief that unless the thought is carried through in the form of a ritual, or compulsion, then something bad will happen. It may start like the avoidance of cracks in the pavement phenomenon, or it may involve touching things. In the latter example this is often associated with a number of times the process has to be gone through. For example, one may feel compelled to touch cutlery ten times before lifting it. Similarly, checking represents another example, whereby an individual might feel compelled to check that the taps in the bathroom are switched off, or that every electrical appliance in the house has been removed, before leaving the home. This checking may then have to be repeated several times so that the individual can literally spend hours chained to the home before leaving for the shortest of times.

Ritual hand-washing, the problem which Lady Macbeth demonstrated so wonderfully, is really quite common. Indeed, I have known children, young adults and elderly spinsters who have felt so compelled to wash their hands through fear of dirt and germs that they have produced the most devastating problems with dermatitis.

The psychology of fixed ideas

A characteristic feature of a fixed idea, or obsessive thought is that it is difficult for the individual to control, even although it may be recognised as being unreasonable. In addition, such thoughts seem to defy the individual's strongest attempts to get rid of them.

As mentioned earlier, some constitutional types, or personalities are particularly prone to develop fixations. In psychiatric terms such people may be called *anankastic*. They are fastidious, like order and organisation, tend to regard punctuality as a virtue and are apt to have strict views about things. It is generally accepted that some psychological trauma may well tip such individuals into a neurotic state characterised by the development of obsessive-compulsive phenomena.

There seem to be two varieties of fixation. Some people develop *obsessive-ruminative* problems, wherein they are subject to some form of repetitive obsessional thinking – eg, having to build up a picture of an individual's face in their mind. Others are subject to *obsessive-compulsive* problems, wherein they may feel compelled to act out some ritualistic behaviour – eg, having to touch wood, wash hands, etc.

The emotion of guilt is a common underlying reason for developing a fixed idea or fixation. As mentioned in Chapter 5, the psychological defence mechanism of *isolation* can often be unconsciously evoked in order to help the individual deal with feelings which might make him feel guilty. Effectively, the repetitive thought or ritual represents an unconscious attempt to isolate the guilt. For example, someone can become obsessed with the thought of harming someone else, perhaps by attacking them with a knife. Understandably, they may begin to feel guilty so the mind strives to protect them from their guilt by firstly developing a phobia about knives, scissors and all pointed objects. Secondly, because this could be impossible to live with, it can initially be softened by building up a ritual around the sharp objects. Thus, the individual may feel that it becomes OK to touch or use a knife, as long as they have stroked the handle twenty times. The problem is that there may follow an escalation so that the twenty times become a hundred times, and so on.

The problem is that frustration is common if the ritual cannot be carried out to perfection for some reason or another. The individual will not be able to accept a 'near-enough' attempt. Any failure to do it properly seems to be 'punishable by the unconscious' with the onset of phobic fear or an acute panic attack.

Sometimes the fixation is a single manifestation in neat, fastitious types, eg *Arsenicum album* or *Nux vomica*, and sometimes it is a symptom in a more deep-rooted problem. Indeed, some 20 per cent of people with troublesome fixations are also depressed.

Guilt

Virtually all of the psychological defence mechanisms mentioned in Chapter 5 can be evoked in order to protect against guilt or potential guilt feelings. Thus, when they work the individual probably has no feeling of guilt. Sometimes, however, the emotion of guilt is so strong that the individual is completely aware of feeling guilty, yet can do nothing to rid themself of the emotion.

The following remedies can be useful when there is consciousness of the emotion of guilt:-

Arsenicum album – for guilt in fussy, fastidious, restless types. If they perceive that they have caused an injury, a slight or a wrong they are liable to suffer anguish out of proportion to the cause. They will be unable to settle and may sink into a deeper anxiety state.

Aurum metallicum – for guilt in depressive types who are prone to take guilt feelings upon themselves. They tend to be self-deprecating and may have self-destructive, or suicidal thoughts. They do, however, fear death. They are particularly sensitive to noise and excitement.

Belladonna – for acute states of guilt, when the individual is suddenly ill. Even forgotten wrongs may flood into the mind and produce intense feelings of guilt.

Causticum – for guilt after shock or bereavement. They feel intensely sympathetic for others, but thinking about their own problems is liable to make the guilt worse. They need to be distracted, because they fear that they have failed everyone.

Cocculus – for guilt in capricious, dreamy types. They can become profoundly sad. They agonise over the health of others and may feel guilty that they have caused the problem. They are worse for movement and often complain of a strange hollowness, or emptiness.

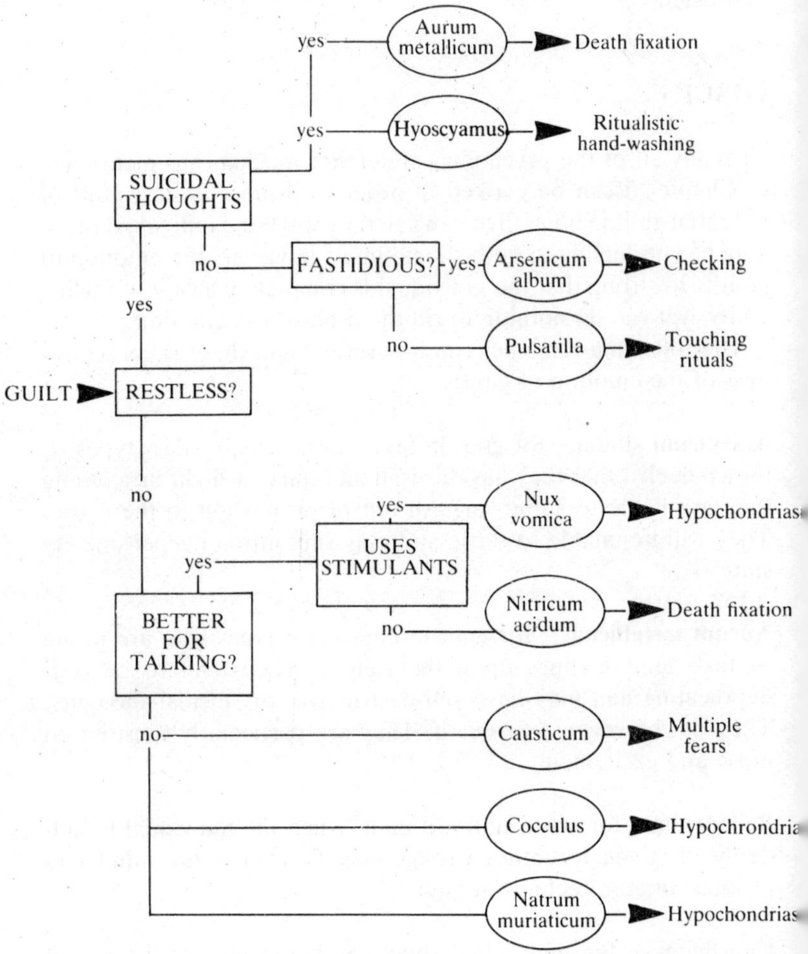

GUILT

Coffea – for guilt in impressionable types. They are quick-thinkers and this is part of their problem. They will agonise about guilt feelings and suffer sleep problems as a result.

Graphites – for guilt in depressive, timid, fidgety types who tend to be overweight. They start or jump at the slightest thing and become weepy on hearing music. Curiously, they may feel as if they sometimes have a cobweb hanging across their face.

Hyoscyamus – for guilt in suspicious, talkative, immodest types. They tend to laugh at inconsequential things. They have a fear of being poisoned or bitten by dogs.

Ignatia – for guilt in introspective, changeable types. They can easily become hysterical. They are generally melancholic and prefer to be silent. They often sigh and sob. They are particularly affected after bereavement.

Natrum muriaticum – for guilt in melancholic types who are worse for consolation. They crave salty foods. They may feel guilty and depressed for a long time after a bereavement or shock.

Nitricum acidum – for guilt in headstrong, irritable, prickly types. Vindictiveness is a characteristic.

Nux vomica – for guilt in fiery, fastidious types who may be high-achievers. They tend to use stimulants, which may make their guilt worse.

Pulsatilla – for guilt in timid, weepy, changeable types who are better for being outdoors. They may feel intensely guilty, yet bottle it all up.

Veratrum album – for guilt in melancholic, indifferent types who are suffering from shock. They will have cold perspiration collecting on their brow.

Fixed Ideas and Fixations

WHERE A FIXATION IS TAKING OVER AN INDIVIDUAL'S LIFE THEY SHOULD ALWAYS CONSULT A DOCTOR.

IF A FIXED IDEA SEEMS COMPLETELY IRRATIONAL AND THE INDIVIDUAL CANNOT APPRECIATE THIS THEN THEY SHOULD BE ENCOURAGED TO CONSULT A DOCTOR, SINCE IT MAY HERALD A MORE SERIOUS EMOTIONAL ILLNESS.

Simple fixed ideas may be helped by the following remedies.

Aconite – after a fright or shock there may be a tendency to fixate upon something. There is often a fear of death and a sense of impending doom. Commonly develop a fixation about not being able to cross the street.

Anacardium orientale – for people who have very bizarre fixations. They may believe that they are two people. They are suspicious, absent-minded and tend to swear. A good remedy for obsessive behaviour in the elderly.

Argentum nitricum – for people prone to all sorts of impulsive actions. They feel compelled because of reasons they are embarrassed to talk about. (See Chapter 4 on Vulnerable Constitutions.)

Arsenicum album – for people who tend to be fussy, tidy and restless. They like everything to be in its place and neatly organised. Very prone to checking.

Aurum metallicum – for fixed ideas in melancholic, self-depreciating types. They become obsessed with death and may have suicidal ideas about how to do it. Nonetheless, they have a great fear of death.

Cuprum metallicum – for morose people with a tendency to spitefulness. They can get very fixed, strange ideas. They usually have a metallic, coppery taste in the mouth and suffer from spasms and cramps.

Hyoscyamus – for fear of water, being bitten, or poisoned. Tendency to develop ritualistic hand-washing. They like things to be arranged symmetrically.

Ignatia – for 'hysterical' types, particularly after shocks or bereavement. May find it difficult to get a face or person out of their mind. May find themselves having to paint a picture of the person in their mind's eye. Tend to be sensitive, weepy and very changeable.

Lachesis – for talkative, suspicious types with a tendency to feel bloated. May develop a religious or philosophical fixation.

Phosphorus – for artistic, creative types who may develop a fixation about health. They fear incurable disease. They fear being suffocated. They may tend to get bleeding disorders, eg, nose-bleeds.

Pulsatilla – for weepy, timid types who are better for sympathy. They fear the opposite sex and may develop very fixed ideas and notions. They may develop rituals about touching wood, etc.

Rhus toxicodendron – for melancholic, restless types with a rheumatic tendency. They may develop a fixation about being poisoned.

Sepia – for indifferent types who come alive when doing a favourite exercise, eg, dancing. They may develop a fixation about disease.

Silicea – for people who are easily discouraged. They dislike mental exertion and may get fixed ideas about small objects like pins. They feel compelled to collect and count them.

Sulphur – for dominant types who find it hard to stay still. They lean, lounge and slouch. They may get a fixation about their body and will scratch and pick, often creating an ear, nose, toe or skin problem as a result.

Tarentula hispania – for those subject to rapidly changing moods. There is a continual pressure to keep busy. May develop fixations about things they dislike and feel compelled to destroy them.

Thuja occidentalis – for hurried, emotionally sensitive types who may be prone to develop warts and polyps. They often have strange fixed ideas, as if their soul and body is separated, or as if they have someone by their side, or as if they have a live animal inside them.

Veratrum album – for melancholic types who may have episodes of hyperactivity and mania. They develop fixations about tearing and cutting things up.

HYPOCHONDRIASIS

Fixations about health, bodily processes, and fear of one's own mortality are all very common. Sometimes the fixation is part of the individual's make-up, their constitution, and sometimes it develops during a flareup of anxiety or depression.

In anxiety states, the fixation may be a secondary effect based upon one of the physical manifestations of their fear. For example, if one experiences palpitations, then the worry about having a weak heart can develop.

In depression, the fixation is likely to be with serious illness. For example, with having cancer, a degenerative or crippling illness. If these sorts of fear are present, then a medical consultation should be sought quickly in order to clear the mind.

The following remedies may be of value.

Arsenicum album – for fussy, tidy types who become quite restless and agitated. When things are not going well they may imagine the worst. They may despair of ever getting better and they may doubt the efficacy or usefulness of any medicine. They may end up pacing the floor at night. They may fear death.

Aurum metallicum – for melancholic, self-depreciating types. They become obsessed with death and may have suicidal thoughts about how to do it. Nonetheless, they have a great fear of death.

Calcarea carbonica – for slow, congested types who have a great fear of mental collapse. They may be in terror of losing their sanity.

Ignatia – for hysterical types who may react to grief, shock or other strong emotions by developing a fixation about their health.

The tendency is part of their makeup. Their reactions are prone to be hysterical.

Natrum muriaticum – for melancholic types who are worse for consolation. They crave salty foods. They are prone to severe headaches.

Nux vomica – for fiery, irritable types who may be high-achievers. They tend to use stimulants and are prone to stomach problems. They may become quite angry as they dwell on their own health.

Valerian – for changeable, over-sensitive types. They may be prone to spasmic pains, flatulence and tremulousness.

CHAPTER 9

Sadness and Depression

In sooth I know not why I am so sad;
It wearies me; you say it wearies you;
But how I caught it, found it, or came by it,
What stuff 'tis made of, whereof it is born
I am to learn;
And such a want-wit sadness makes of me,
That I have much ado to know myself.

William Shakespeare,
The Merchant of Venice

Sadness and depression are extremely common. Although the two words have a similar meaning, they are generally thought of as having a different significance. Whereas most people feel sad on occasions, it is thought that a smaller number suffer from the more severe state of depression. In fact there is no real consensus opinion, because psychiatrists disagree upon the nature of depression itself.

Some psychiatrists consider that sadness merely represents the milder end of the range of an emotion, with suicidal depression at the other end. Others would write sadness off as a temporary normal state, to be differentiated from the definite illnesses of depression. In the latter case they would distinguish between neurotic depression and the psychotic affective disorders, eg manic-depressive psychosis and psychotic depression.

To complicate matters further, there is considerable debate as to whether depression is physically or psychologically based. This is illustrated in the way depression is still differentiated into the so-called *endogenous* and *reactive* types of depression. It has to be said that this is no longer used as a strict classification, yet it undoubtedly still serves as the model which many psychiatrists use to decide upon treatment.

Endogenous depression is thought to arise as a result of some genetic or biochemical problem. It is classically associated with sleep disturbance (usually early morning waking), loss of appetite, loss of sex drive, constipation and perhaps even indigestion.

Reactive depression is thought to arise from some obvious emotional trauma or loss. It is less likely to be associated with the so-called 'biological features' of depression.

The significance of differentiating the two is that endogenous types of depression are thought to be more likely to respond to drugs and physical methods of treatment. On the other hand, reactive depressions are more likely to respond to psychotherapeutic methods of treatment, the simplest of all being reassurance.

The truth of the matter, however, is that it is rarely possible to be specific. Most cases of depression have mixed features, which means that there are probably multiple reasons for the depression, as well as differing perceptions of the way the individual feels depressed.

Indeed, it is because people react in an individual manner when they feel sad or depressed that homoeopathy has so much to offer.

The main features of sadness and depression

Before looking at individual remedies it is as well to consider features which occur relatively commonly in depression.

*lowness in spirits
*loss of vitality
*feelings of guilt
*self-depreciation
*hopelessness and despair
*sleep disturbance
*variation in mood throughout the day

The problems are that once one sinks into a state of depression there may be great difficulty in looking ahead. The future may seem black and gloomy, or there may seem to be no future to look forward to at all.

Guilt feelings are often quite unjustifiable, yet are difficult to get rid of. They can produce further self-depreciation and a sense of being useless to anyone. The danger here is that the individual may contemplate self-harm or suicide.

IF THERE ARE ANY THOUGHTS OF SELF-HARM OR SUICIDE THEN MEDICAL HELP SHOULD BE SOUGHT URGENTLY.

Homoeopathy and depression

As mentioned above depression can be extremely dangerous if the individual loses their sense of hope. Quite simply, if life loses its appeal then a suicidal attempt may follow. For this reason if the depression is severe or is slow to lift, conventional help is always essential.

It is also important that the individual SHOULD NEVER STOP TAKING CONVENTIONAL MEDICATION EXCEPT UPON MEDICAL ADVICE. Having said that, homoeopathic remedies can be taken alongside conventional treatment with good results.

As mentioned in Chapter 4, certain constitutional types are vulnerable to depression. If the constitutional remedy is easily spotted, then this should be taken at the start of any episode of low spirits, to prevent the depression taking hold.

Also, as mentioned in Chapter 5, many people may protect themselves by encapsulating their depression within another emotion. If this is the case, then it is as well to aim the treatment at the type of depression, rather than at the second (or third) emotion.

Agitated Depression

Restlessness is the dominant feature in these types of reaction. There may be irritability, fidgeting, pacing and a want to hurry everything.

Arsenicum album – for sadness and depression in fussy, tidy, generally restless types. They fall into bouts of deep anguish. They will fidget and pace the floor. They will despair of ever being well and will doubt the effectiveness of treatments.

Aurum metallicum – for sudden onset of sadness or depression almost descending like a cloud. Feels worthless, despondent about everything and disgusted with self and life. May feel suicidal, although fears death. Cannot keep still or be quiet.

Belladonna – for sudden onset of sadness and depression. Speed of onset and the type of accompanying physical reaction are characteristic. The pupils may seem dilated, the cheeks hot and suffused and the pulse bounding. They will be restless and 'pumped up.'

Iodum – for sadness and depression when the future seems dim. Cannot settle and gets impulses to run away and do destructive, aggressive acts. Shuns company and may think about self-harm or suicide.

Lilium tigrinum – for restless sadness and depression in weepy, anxious types, mainly females. May suffer from premenstrual syndrome. Tendency to indifference. Has to keep busy, but without any real aim.

Natrum muriaticum – for sadness and depression in types who can fly into a passion over trivia, are worse for consolation and who love salt. They can become awkward, hasty and restless.

Nitricum acidum – for sadness and depression in prickly, irritable types. They sink into despair, but can become quite vindictive and 'prickly.' They are very sensitive to all things.

Nux vomica – for irritable, restless depression and sadness. May be a high achiever who feels that they have let things slip by them. Can be very fiery when pressed. May suffer from digestive problems.

Phosphorus – for artistic, creative types who tend to have bouts of sadness. They are fidgety and restless. They constantly need reassurance.

Rhus toxicodendron – for sadness and depression with extreme restlessness. They cannot keep still for a moment. They are worse at night and cannot stay in bed. Tendency to suffer from rheumatic problems. Fears of being poisoned.

Lethargic or Retarded Depression

Lethargy and slowness of movement, thought and reduced concentration are the characteristics of these reactions.

Calcarea carbonica – for sadness and depression in slow, worrying types who are prone to congestive problems. They are worse for even slight mental and physical exertion.

China officinalis – for sadness and depression especially after blood loss or loss of body fluids, eg, after a diarrhoeal illness. Although they feel depressed and lethargic, however, their minds will be positively 'buzzing.'

Graphites – for sadness and depression in timid, indecisive types. They are generally apprehensive about things, startle easily and may complain of a curious cob-web sensation over the face.

Kali phosphoricum – for sadness in anxious types who have a dread of meeting people. When depressed they slip into complete lethargy and may find their memory deteriorates. They may sleep-walk and suffer from nightmares and night terrors.

Sepia – for sadness and depression in indifferent types who seem to come alive when doing a favourite thing, eg, dancing. Worse for sympathy and company, yet dreads being left to their own devises.

Sulphur – for sadness and depression in dominant, selfish types. They tend to lean, slouch and lounge and always find it difficult to motivate themselves, especially when feeling sad. Never quite manage to look smart.

Veratrum album – for sadness and depression with great exhaustion. Tendency to perspire over the brow. Seems indifferent to everything. Has desire to tear and cut things up.

Hysterical Depression

The characteristic reaction here is of sudden impulsive, theatrical gestures. There may be desperate sighs, bouts of loud crying, sudden outbursts of temper and rapid changes of mood. When depressed there may be self-destructive or suicidal gestures. There may be the prima donna extroverted personality, or the apparent introvert who is able to don the theatre mask which allows them to play the part of the extrovert.

Cimicifuga – for primadonna-ish depression with dreams of impending evil. Talks all the time and may make self-destructive gestures. Completely unpredictable hysterical outbursts.

Ignatia – for hysterical depression in changeable, introspective types. Dramatic sighing and weeping. Particularly prone after shocks and bereavements.

Lachesis – for sadness in talkative, suspicious types prone to bloating. Likes to escape from problems. Can be very jealous and dramatic in reactions.

Pulsatilla – for hysterical depression in timid, weepy types who prefer the outdoors. They are better for sympathy. Fear the opposite sex. They will weep at all sorts of things, eg, romantic films, music etc. Sometimes they will use their tears to good advantage.

Valerian – for hysterical depression in over-sensitive, irritable types with a changeable nature. Tendency to be very shaky and with a proneness to spasms of all sorts.

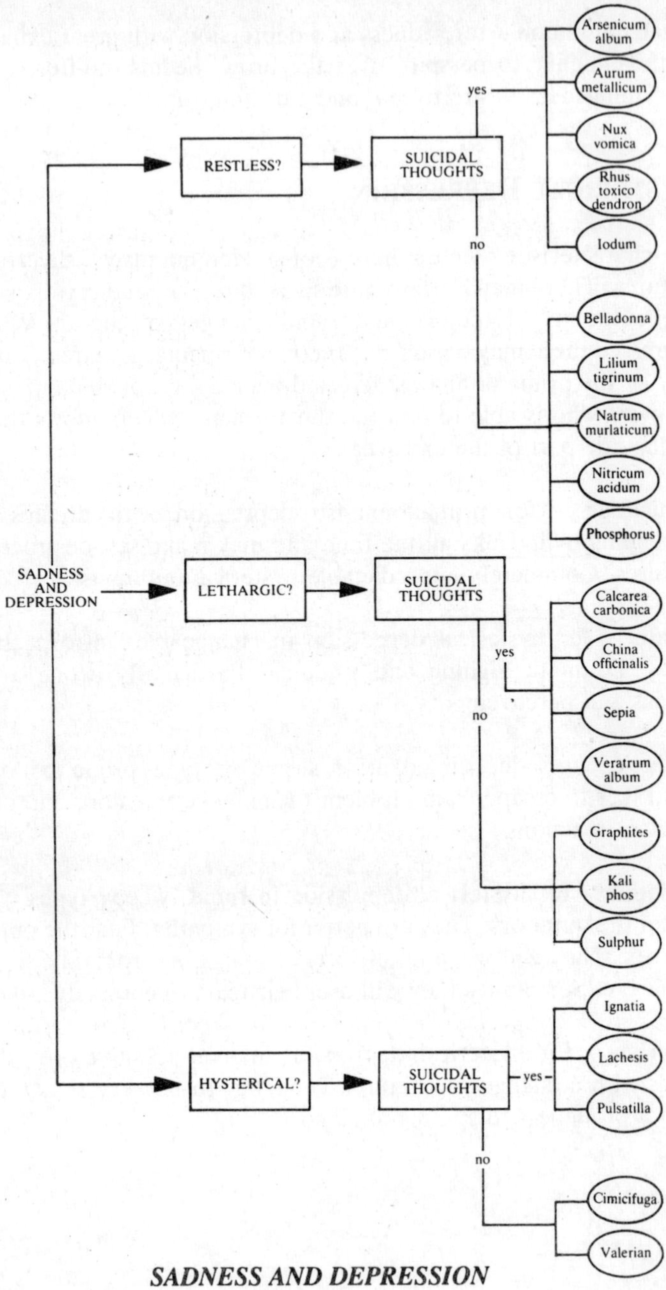

SADNESS AND DEPRESSION

TEARFULNESS

The tendency to weep varies from person to person. For example, some people weep easily, under any circumstances, whereas other can only weep when they are alone.

And people may weep for different reasons. Some might only ever weep when profoundly depressed, while others can feel the tears welling up when they are happy, sad or on the point of rage.

Apis mellifica – for tearfulness in indifferent, apathetic types. May suffer very sensitive, piercing pains, when tend to shriek. There is whining with the tearfulness.

Ignatia – for tearfulness in hysterical types. Reactions always tend to be over the top. Useful for the reaction in grief.

Natrum muriaticum – for tearfulness in melancholic types who are worse for consolation. They will always try to be on their own in order to let the tears come.

Pulsatilla – for timid, weepy types who are generally better for consolation. Prefer to be outdoors.

Rhus toxicodendron – for melancholic, listless types, prone to rheumatic problems. They are always better for limbering-up or moving around.

Sepia – for indifferent types who may be quite irritable and easily offended. They are generally better if they can be persuaded to do some favourite physical activity.

CHAPTER 10

Grief and Bereavement

Can I see another's woe,
And not be in sorrow too?
Can I see another's grief,
And not seek for kind relief?

William Blake,
On Another's Sorrow

Grief is something which most people can expect to experience at some stage of their life. It is the price we pay for forging attachments, friendships and relationships. Because we grow close to people, like them and love them, we miss them when they are gone.

There is a general sequence of observed stages of grief common to most people. After a bereavement, the individual may go through three stages of grief:-

1) *Protective numbness and shock*, usually lasting a week or two. This may allow the individual to cope with funeral arrangements and the funeral itself.

2) *Intense grief and distress*, usually lasting 6 to 12 weeks. During this stage the individual may experience emotions such as anger, guilt, developing depression and fear. There may be a tendency to bottle things up, have outbursts of irritability or rage, or episodes of hysteria.

3) *Constant depression*, lasting for another 6 to 12 weeks.

Following this is the resolution, or recovery which may take one or two years. It is the time when the pain fades and the emotional wound starts to heal. All of this represents normal grief.

'Atypical grief,' on the other hand, is characterised by abnormal length of the stages, or by particularly intense reactions. There may be excessive guilt, profound depression and even suicidal thoughts. IF THERE IS ANY SUGGESTION OF ATYPICAL GRIEF WITH SUICIDAL THOUGHTS, A MEDICAL OPINION SHOULD BE SOUGHT URGENTLY.

Homoeopathy and grief

Although the stages of grief are well documented, the experience of grief is unique to the individual. While there may be similarities in the progression of emotions, the way the individual reacts will be personal to them. Since homoeopathy aims at treating the individual reaction, it is an ideal method for taking the edge off the emotions. If appropriate remedies are selected the grieving process can be gone through with less pain, and in a shorter time. Also, if dealt with quickly enough there is less chance of normal grief developing into the more sinister and dangerous 'atypical grief.'

The following remedies are useful.

Arsenicum album – for grief when there is marked restlessness. The individual cannot settle, needs constant consoling and may become full of fear.

Aurum metallicum – for grief when there is excessive guilt, self-depreciation, profound depression and possible suicidal thoughts. They may feel extremely sensitive to noise. They may develop an illness through the grief.

Causticum – for grief when the individual seems very sympathetic and caring about others around them. The more they think about their own grief, the worse they feel, so they are better when distracted. They may develop an illness through the grief.

Ignatia – for grief when the individual seems changeable, possibly with hysterical outbursts. May feel very guilty. May have headaches, like a nail being driven into the skull. May develop an

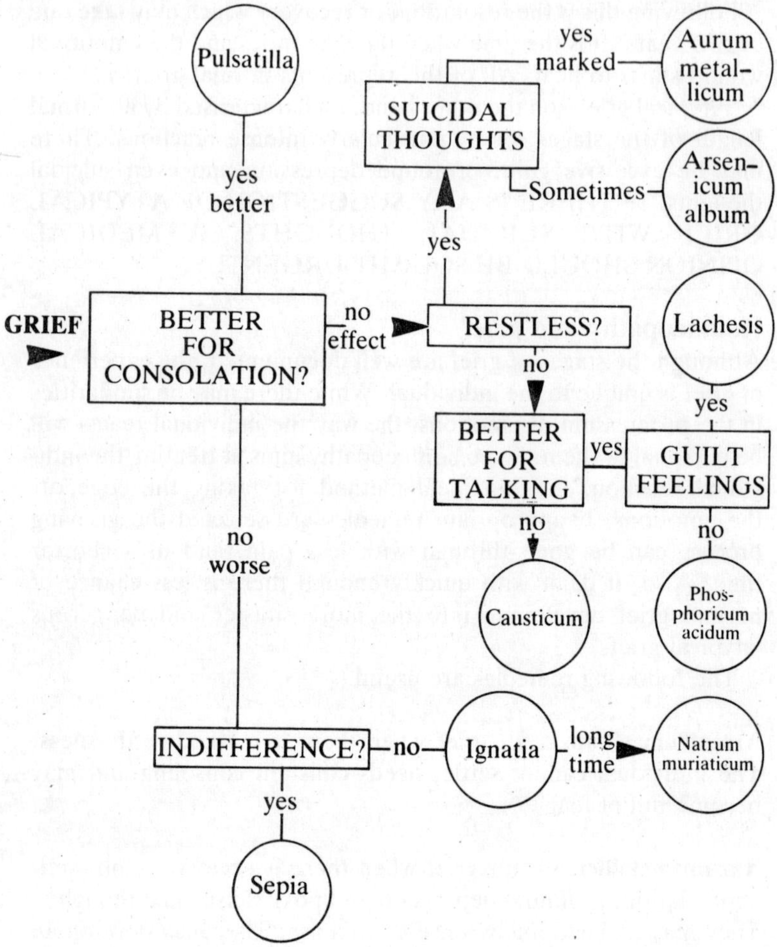

GRIEF

illness through the grief. Probably the best remedy to be taken in the first stage of grief.

Lachesis – for grief in talkative, excitable types with a tendency to feel bloated. May become quite jealous of people round about. May envy those who have not lost their loved ones, or may even feel jealous of the departed for some reason. May develop illness through the grief.

Natrum muriaticum – for grief in melancholic, touchy types. They are worse for consolation, so may become quite reclusive in bereavement. Alternatively, they may seem to become aloof. Both are means of avoiding consolation. It is very appropriate when depression becomes marked. Generally, likes salt and salty things.

Phosphoric acid – for grief in mild, indifferent types. They become quite exhausted and tangled in their thoughts. They become quite despairing and may be exhausted and depressed for a long time.

Pulsatilla – for grief in weepy, timid, changeable types who prefer to be outdoors. They need company, someone to talk to, and they are better for consolation.

Sepia – for grief in melancholic, indifferent types. They are very weepy, dislike sympathy, yet want people to be somewhere near – although not in the same room. May feel that they want to run away from it all.

CHAPTER 11

Anger and Irritability

Anger is one of the sinews of the soul
Thomas Fuller (1608–1661)

Anger is one of the emotions which has a marked physical component. Many of the old sayings exemplify this – people go 'red with rage,' or 'white with fury;' they feel their 'blood boil,' or their 'bile rise;' or they may seem to go 'apoplectic,' 'mad,' or 'frenzied.'

Interestingly, these expressions vary in age and origin. Some are relatively recent, reflecting the medical concern about anger causing a rise in blood pressure leading to an apoplectic attack or stroke. The bloated, suffused face is thus taken as a danger signal that the individual might 'burst a blood vessel.'

Other expressions reflect a feeling that the blood is heating up. Of course, the temperature of the blood does not actually change. Such expressions are mere analogies, in that they describe the sense of mounting anger, relating it to the speed and intensity with which a liquid boils. Similarly, going 'blind with fury,' does not imply any actual visual loss, but means that the angered individual is unable to focus on anything except his anger.

Finally, expressions about bile are mediaeval in origin, referring as they do to the belief that bile was one of the four humours, or vital fluids. It was held that if the humour became excessive, then anger resulted. Not only that, but if the anger persisted without relief, then illness would result. Indeed, as we shall see later, the suppression of anger can cause illness in some people.

The behavioural component can also be quite marked. People

are known to 'shake,' 'seethe,' 'tremble,' 'shake fists,' or 'go dangerously quiet.'

Often the expression of anger can be a matter of degree, with slight irritability at one end of the range and blind fury at the other. It is also true to say that some people react in a way which is characteristic of them as individuals. Some may only ever get slightly irritable, while others react in an explosive sort of way with no intermediate stages of arousal or warning.

As mentioned in Chapter 4, some people have irritable constitutions or natures. They are never far from being tipped into anger. For example, the Nux vomica constitution is irritable, quarrelsome, and will tend to flare into a tantrum when contradicted. These outbursts are part of the inate coping mechanism of the Nux vomica constitution.

Other types feel the anger building within them, yet have coping mechanisms to 'let the steam off.'

Unfortunately, other people are like boilers with faulty safety valves. Sometimes their coping mechanisms work, but at other times they fail and the pressure continues to build up until a critical point is reached. A seemingly inappropriate behavioural reaction may result, eg, the normally placcid type flying off the handle, or becoming violent. Alternatively, psychological defence mechanisms (See Chapter 5) suppress the emotion, with the later development of illness.

Coping

There are many time-honoured ways of coping with anger, from the 'hold your breath and count to ten' approach, to the 'go home and kick the cat' method. Some people find that they are better for hitting a hundred golf balls, others from having a good shout, and still others from breaking a few plates.

The people who most need to establish coping mechanisms, I feel, are the types who bottle up their anger and become ill. They may even be doing this because they fear 'letting go,' since they are aware of having a violent temper. While they may not be doing anyone harm by internalising their problem, they may be putting themselves at risk of heart disease, bowel problems and possibly even malignant disease.

I do not advocate any single coping technique for such people, because I feel that the technique must fit the individual. For example, people who are not good at verbalising are unlikely to feel better for making themselves rant and rave, but they may feel better for doing something physical to some inanimate object, eg, beating a drum, digging the garden or chopping wood.

Again, it is all about 'knowing yourself.'

IRRITABILITY

The following remedies are useful when there is over-sensitivity, irritability over minor problems and a dislike of being contradicted.

Anacardium orientale – when there is extreme over-sensitivity in someone with a poor memory. They may become abusive and malicious. They often have peculiar fixations.

Arsenicum album – when there is restlessness and irritability in a fussy, fastidious type of person.

Aurum metallicum – when there is irritability in someone given to sudden severe bouts of depression, with feelings of self-depreciation. Markedly over-sensitive.

Belladonna – for irritability when suddenly ill, with a flushed appearance and a bounding pulse.

Bryonia – for extreme irritability, especially when 'everything is wrong.' All symptoms are worse for movement.

Capsicum – classically a 'peppery' type. Doesn't like to go far from home, but likes solitude. A good remedy for homesickness.

Chamomilla – for irritability in children and those in the Third Age. Whining, over-sensitive, impatient and snappy.

Cina officinalis – for irritability and peevishness. Not happy even when they get their own way. Variable appetite. Tendency to suffer from spasmodic pains.

Colocynth – for irritability and extreme dislike of being contradicted. Indignation about personal slights.

Hepar sulph – for irritability in melancholic types who are better in damp weather. Irritable at the slightest things. May be violent when angered.

Ignatia – for irritability in people of changeable, hysterical nature.

Lachesis – for irritability in talkative, jealous, melancholic types with a tendency to feel bloated. Can be a bit like *Dr Jekyll and Mr Hyde* in their reactions – especially in women premenstrually (See Chapter 16). May say deliberately hurtful things.

Lycopodium – for irritability in worried, professional types. They tend to suffer anticipatory anxiety and dislike criticism

Natrum muriaticum – for irritability in melancholic types who are worse for consolation. They can fly into a passion over trivia.

Nitricum acidum – for irritability in 'prickly' types. They can be vindictive when crossed. They are over-sensitive to everything. They are usually very stubborn. They have a tendency to suffer from ulcers and blisters, and all pains 'prickle' or are 'splinter-like.'

Nux vomica – for irritability in over-sensitive 'fiery' types. They are always finding fault with others and do not see their own short-comings. They tend to rely on stimulants.

Phosphorus – for irritability and dislike of criticism in artistic, creative types who may feel clairvoyant. They have a tendency towards bleeding disorders.

Platina – for irritability in extremely arrogant types. Physical symptoms tend to disappear when they get mental symptoms. Tremulousness is common. Everything has to be done in a hurry.

Pulsatilla – for irritability and peevishness in weepy, changeable types who are generally better for being outdoors.

Sepia – for irritability in indifferent, melancholic types. If they can be encouraged to do some favourite activity, eg, dancing, they may 'come alive.'

Staphisagria – for irritability and peevishness in those who are over-sensitive to criticism. They may be impulsive and aggressive when angered. Alternatively, they may bottle things up.

Thuja occidentalis – for irritability in those who are subject to fixed ideas (See Chapter 8). They may become quite weepy. Tend to suffer from warty problems and have a great fondness for tea.

Anger and Rage

Although all of the preceding remedy-profiles are useful in irritability and anger, the following are particularly good if there are outbursts of severe rage.

Aconite – for acute flare-ups of anger after an accident or shock.

Belladonna – for sudden 'blowing of the top' – literally like a volcano, with redness and a feeling of rising heat.

Chamomilla – for sudden outbursts in children and those in the Third Age. There is an underlying snappy, over-sensitive nature.

Hepar sulph – for sudden violent behaviour, even with the desire to maime or kill, in an irritable person who is generally better for damp weather. May be verbally abusive.

Ignatia – for sudden hysterical outbursts of anger in changeable, irritable, hysterical people.

Nux vomica – for sudden outbursts of anger in irritable, tetchy types who tend to use stimulants. May be vicious. Hate being contradicted.

Sepia – for unexpected anger, as if something suddenly snaps, in usually indifferent, melancholic types. Particularly so if premenstrual or menopausal.

Staphisagria – for sudden violent outbursts in types who feel anger, but usually bottle it up.

Sulphur – for anger and aggression in dominant types who find it hard to look smart. May be the 'ragged philosopher' type who becomes incensed by injustice.

Illness after Anger

As mentioned earlier, it has been observed many times in history that persisting, or suppressed anger can cause illness.

All sorts of ailments can be caused, but common ones are associated with the following remedies.

Apis mellifica – for skin or mouth problems, with puffiness, swelling and stinging after anger.

Bryonia – for rheumatic problems which are worse for movement, in irritable types after anger.

Chamomilla – for diarrhoeal illness, insomnia and exquisitely painful and sensitive problems (eg, toothache, earache) in irritable types. They react to their ailments in an angry manner, just as the ailments can occur if they become angry.

Colocynth – for abdominal colic, neuralgia and sciatica when angry, or following 'swallowed anger.' Classically causes left-sided problems.

Gelsemium – for episodes of vertigo, trembling and even bouts of paralysis after anger. Generally quiet types who prefer to be left to themselves.

Ignatia – for difficulty in swallowing after suppressed anger. May find it difficult to swallow food, especially in public, leading to the development of a social phobia.

Lycopodium – for stomach and digestive problems after suppression of anger. Tend to be professional types who are prone to worry about performing in public.

Nux vomica – for 'liverish' and digestive problems in tetchy, irritable types who tend to like good food, wine and use stimulants. Very sensitive. May have problems with hernias.

Phosphoricum acidum – for general debility, exhaustion, eye problems and nose-bleeds in generally mild types who suppress their anger.

Stramonium – for skin and throat problems in those types who suppress their temper tantrums.

Staphisagria – for headaches, warts, polyps, bladder and urinary problems in impatient types who swallow their anger, because they know that they have a violent temper.

CHAPTER 12

Love, Hate and Jealousy

I hate and I love: why I do so you may well ask. I do not know, but I feel it happen and am in agony.

Catullus (87–54 BC)

It is said that love makes the world go round. It has also been said that hate keeps it spinning. The sheer power of these emotions have been recognised since the beginnings of time.

It is probably true to say that love is the most unfathomable of the emotions. The Ancient Greeks, those masters at encapsulating sentiments and emotions into the form of great deities, made the goddess Aphrodite the very essence of love.

The name *Aphrodite* (Venus to the Romans), was probably of oriental origin. It is likely that she was derived from the earlier Assyro-Babylonian goddess *Ishtar*, a voluptuous warrior deity, and the Syro-Phoenician goddess *Astarte*, patron deity of orgies. The spread of the various cults and the amalgamation of one into another would have been inevitable in those dim and distant days when one maritime power traded, fought and overcame another.

And so Aphrodite came to be venerated throughout the Aegean. But just as today we recognise different types of love, so too was Aphrodite known by different names in different centres according to the character of the love which was being represented. Thus, *Aphrodite Urania*, the celestial Aphrodite, was the goddess of pure or ideal love. *Aphrodite Genetrix* or *Nymphia*, was the protector of marriages. *Aphrodite Porne*, was the goddess of lust and the patroness of prostitutes. Finally, *Aphrodite Anosia* (the impious) was the goddess of unfaithful lovers. She was the mistress of gracious laughter, sweet deceits, the charms and delights of love.

Not only was Aphrodite worshipped, but she had a retinue of other deities who loved her, followed her or supposedly had played important parts in her 'life.' Among these was *Eros*, (Cupid to the Romans) a beautiful winged deity who fired arrows from a golden quiver at unsuspecting mortals. The effect was instant love and passion, as if the wounded party had been smitten in the heart.

Another was *Psyche* (meaning the soul). According to legend she was a maiden of such beauty that Aphrodite herself became jealous. In order to teach the mortal a lesson she sent Eros to punish her. As it happened, Eros fell in love with her and visited her nightly, until her two sisters urged her to discover his identity. Eros left her and she went though agonies as she tried to recapture her lost love. For Aphrodite's part, jealousy deepened to become the bitterest hatred.

This little aside into the realms of Ancient Greek mythology is fairly instructive. It shows that there are many different types of love, and that pride, jealousy and bitterness can all be somehow related in the dynamics of relationships. Hate, the negative of love, can stem from any of these. Undoubtedly, it is one of the hardest emotions to live with.

Love-Sickness

By this term I refer to those conditions which come about through unrequited, or disappointed love. They can vary from the loss of interest in life of the proverbially 'heart-broken,' to stress-induced asthma, psychosomatic bowel problems, or even the development of degenerative disease.

Broken relationships, marital breakdowns, family squabbles, all of these can produce problems in the individual beyond the initial trauma. The following remedies may help.

Aurum metallicum – for great depression and possible suicidal thoughts in generally melancholic types.

Calcarea phosphorica – for fretfulness, skin problems, vertigo, migraine and rheumatic problems after unrequited love. Will be worse the more that they think about the problem. Are better on their own, although cannot settle and will move from room to room.

Causticum – for illness or ailments after disappointed or unrequited love in over-sensitive types who will always be sympathetic for others. They may even have sympathy for the other party in the relationship or squabble. They may develop bladder problems, insomnia, or wart problems.

Cimicifuga – for depression and the feeling that a cloud of impending doom has descended after an unsuccessful romance. May develop painful conditions in which the pains feel like electric shocks. Women often develop gynaecological problems.

Coffea – for insomnia, headaches like a 'nail being driven into the skull,' and 'mind-buzz' after unsuccessful or unrequited love. Most problems relate to the fact that the person cannot get the problem out of their head.

Hyoscyamus – for severe restlessness, even amounting to fits after a disappointing love affair. May become jealous, suspicious, angry. May want to break or tear things up – love letters, for example.

Ignatia – for hysterical reactions to disappointed love. May become very emotional, but rapidly changeable. May develop difficulty in swallowing after such a problem.

Lachesis – for angry outbursts and jealousy after disappointed love in talkative types with a tendency to become bloated. Are prone to Premenstrual Syndrome. (See separate Chapter.)

Natrum muriaticum – for the development of ailments like migraine with zig-zag vision, depression, palpitations and skin problems, after disappointed love in melancholic types who are worse for consolation. They crave salt or salty foods.

Nux vomica – for stomach and digestive problems following disappointed love in fiery, high-achievers who are prone to over-use stimulants. They hate being contradicted.

Phosphoric acidum – for the ill-effects of disappointed or unrequited love in mild, gentle types. They become very listless and apathetic. They lose interest in everything around them and seem to find difficulty in grasping anything. They may sink into despair.

Sepia – for loss of interest in everything and everybody in people who generally seem indifferent. They hate sympathy, yet dislike being left on their own. They like thunderstorms and seem to come alive if they can be prompted to do some favourite activity, eg, dancing.

Staphisagria – for disappointed love when there are violent outbursts in extremely sensitive types. Pride is a characteristic feature and they may become quite indignant because of the personal slight which they perceive. On the other hand they may bottle their emotion up and become quite ill.

HATE

As mentioned above, hate is one of the hardest emotions to live with. Whereas love is associated with the heart, hate has been associated with the soul. When it persists for long enough it can almost literally seem to eat away at the soul. All positive emotions become forfeit to the unrelenting burning heat of hate.

It is obviously outside the scope of this book to look at the things which can produce hate, but since it is such a strong emotion its effects upon the individual are best countered with the appropriate homoeopathic remedy. By this, I mean the severity of the hate itself, or the development of an ailment when there is a dominant feeling of hate in the emotional life.

Anacardium orientale – for hate in easily offended, hypochondriacal types. They become quite vindictive and malicious in their hate. They often develop odd fixed ideas. Their language may be abusive and strong.

Aurum metallicum – for melancholic types who may feel suicidal. Their hate mechanism seems finely tuned, in that they can hate and loathe people whom they perceive have offended them. It is usually out of proportion to the perceived offence.

Calcarea carbonica – for hate in slow, melancholic, easily exhausted types who have a tendency towards all sorts of congestive problems. They are full of fears. They may grow to hate those who take things out on them, or who shine in comparison to them.

Cuprum metallicum – for hate in those people who get fixed ideas in their mind. They become very malicious and spiteful. If they can even a score they will do so. They tend to suffer from spasms and cramps and have a metallic taste in the mouth.

Lachesis – for hate in talkative, suspicious types with a tendency to feel bloated. They may become quite angry and will look for means of verbally hurting the target of their hatred.

Natrum muriaticum – for hate in melancholic types who are easily offended and tend to hold grudges, often for years. They are worse for consolation. They crave salt or salty foods.

Nitricum acidum – for hate in prickly types who will be spiteful and unforgiving despite apologies from the target of their hatred.

Phosphorus – for hate in creative, artistic types who are very sensitive. They may hold grudges and can flare-up like a match.

Rhus toxicodendron – for hate in restless rheumatic types. Their rheumatic pains may in fact worsen or develop after the onset of their hate.

Sulphur – for hate of institutions and injustice in 'ragged philosopher' types. They find it hard not to slouch, lean or fidget. They make good campaigners if they can channel their emotion and overcome their natural indolent tendency.

Jealousy

> *O! Beware, my lord, of jealousy;*
> *It is the green-eyed monster which doth mock*
> *the meat it feeds on.*
>
> William Shakespeare, *Othello*

The green-eyed monster of jealousy has toppled governments, lost kingdoms and created misery throughout the history of mankind. Those who are afflicted by it can find themselves doing great acts of maliciousness or smaller deeds of spite. It is a completely negative emotion which can cause harm to the individual, as well as to others through the action of the jealous person.

Defining it is extremely difficult. Two of the most famous attempts to do so are:-

> *. . . kind of fear related to a desire to preserve a possession.*
>
> Descartes

and

> *. . . mixture of hate and love.*
>
> Spinoza

When there is a real conscious feeling of jealousy, then the following remedies might help.

Apis mellifica – for those who are afflicted by apathy and indifference. They may feel as if they are about to die and they will feel jealous of people around them. They may feel intensely suspicious of the actions of relatives and spouses. They may be fidgety and subject to sensitive and very painful conditions.

Arsenicum album – for fussy, tidy and restless types. They may find themselves becoming jealous of others who possess neater or more aesthetically refined things than themselves.

Calcarea carbonica – for slow, melancholic types who are prone to all sorts of congestive problems. They are averse to mental and physical exertion, so may under-achieve. Consequently, when they feel depressed in spirits they may become jealous of friends and neighbours who apparently have everything.

Hyoscyamus – for talkative, suspicious types who are immodest with a tendency to expose themselves. They can become very jealous of other people and make fools of themselves through odd behaviour. They may go into fits of laughter about inconsequential things. They may be afraid of being poisoned, so will be suspicious of food, medicines and drinks.

Ignatia – for changeable, impulsive types. They may develop bouts of jealousy after grief or loss. Their reaction may be hysterical.

Lachesis – for talkative, suspicious types with a tendency to feel bloated. They tend to be night owls who work best late at night, but inefficiently early in the day. They may get quite clumsy. They may have fits of temper when jealousy will come out as verbal abuse. The jealousy is particularly likely premenstrually or round about the menopause.

Lycopodium – for worried, highly-strung types who anticipate events with fear. They may envy other people who are able to carry any situation off, while they agonise for days ahead. They tend to be professionals and they may become jealous of their colleagues' attainments or popularity.

Nux vomica – for fiery, irritable types who tend to use stimulants. They are constantly pressured and may become high-achievers. Their jealousy is liable to produce bouts of irritability. They may be jealous of colleagues, partners or other people. They may feel that the grass is always greener on the other side of the fence. They may make themselves ill and develop digestive problems.

Pulsatilla – for timid, weepy types who are better for being outdoors. They have changeable natures and may become extremely jealous quite swiftly. They are, however, quite likely to bottle-up their jealousy.

Staphisagria – for extremely sensitive, easily offended types. Their offended sense of pride may make them prone to jealousy. Their

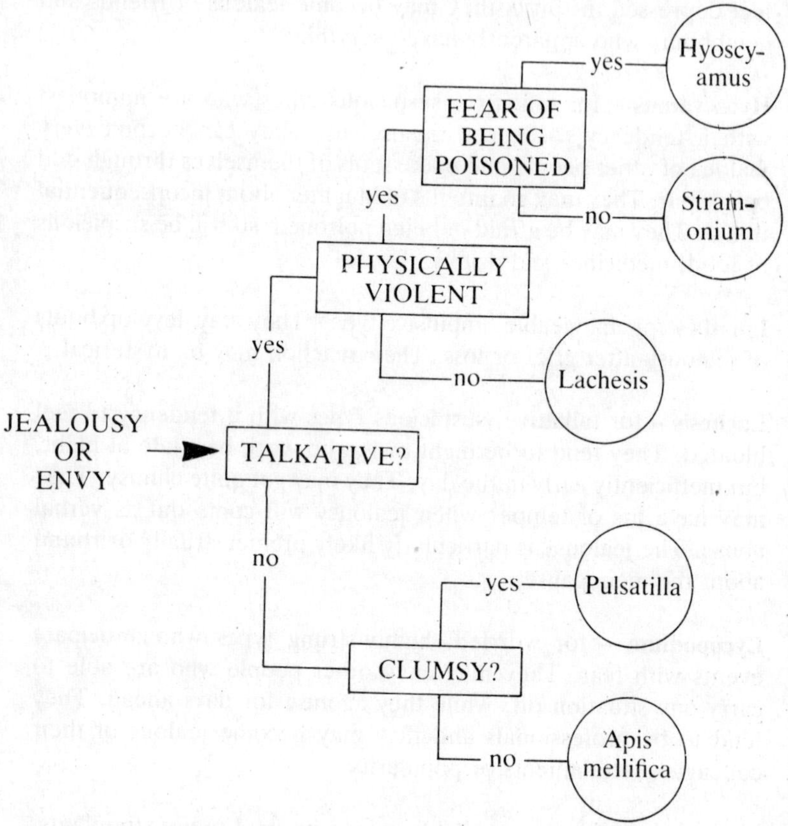

JEALOUSY

reaction could swing towards complete apathy, or a violent outburst of passion. They prefer solitude to company. They may become fixated about sexual problems.

Stramonium – for intense, talkative types. They tend to have rapid mood changes. Their jealousy may seem out of context, as is their reaction. They may become very aggressive and violent.

CHAPTER 13

Exhaustion and Chronic Fatigue

Exhaustion and chronic fatigue have always been common problems in Medicine. In recent years, however, there have been various attempts to label a condition, the characteristics of which are extreme physical and mental fatigue in the absence of any recognised organic problem.

In the 1950s an outbreak of a mysterious debilitating illness took place at the Royal Free Hospital in London. The affected staff were smitten with extreme lassitude, easy muscle fatiguability and troubles with concentration. This became known as Royal Free Disease.

Over the years the same cluster of symptoms have been redescribed under the following names:-

Royal Free Disease
Neuromyasthenia
Icelandic Disease
Post Viral Syndrome
Yuppie Flu
Chronic Mononucleosis (a chronic Glandular Fever)
Effort Syndrome
Myalgic Encephalomyelitis
Chronic Fatigue Syndrome

The problem with many of these names is that they imply a particular pathological process or a particular cause. For example, Post Viral Syndrome implies that it is a state arising after an infection with a virus. The commonest was thought to be influenza or an influenza-like illness. The second commonest was thought to be the Epstein-Barr virus, the agent which causes Infectious Mononucleosis or Glandular Fever.

The newer label of Myalgic Encephalomyelitis, on the other hand, suggests that there is a particular problem affecting the muscles (Myalgic, meaning pain in the muscles) and the brain and nervous system (encephalo, meaning brain; and myelitis, meaning inflammation of the nerves and spinal cord). The problem with this term is that while it may describe what seems to happen, there are no tests which can be done to actually demonstrate that this is the case.

The most recently devised label is Chronic Fatigue Syndrome. It is used because it does not imply any actual physical disorder, but is suggestive of the main complaint, ie, fatigue. So far it seems to be the term most readily accepted by the orthodox medical profession. However, many support groups feel that it is inappropriate, because there seems to be an implication that the condition is mainly psychological.

Whichever of these terms is used, however, it is important to appreciate that it is nothing more than a blanket term. It is, I believe, like diagnosing depression as a single entity, or Rheumatoid Arthritis as a unique physical disease.

The following problems have all been said to occur and be covered by the Chronic Fatigue Syndrome blanket term.

Myalgic Encephalomyelitis
Post Viral Syndrome
Intestinal Candidiasis
Hypoglycaemia
Depression
Multiple Food Allergies

Myalgic Encephalomyelitis Classically, this starts as a sore throat and flu-like illness with enlarged glands. There may be symptoms of diarrhoea and vomiting, dizziness and palpitations. Recovery is slow and extreme fatigue and muscle weakness occur. There are usually problems with memory, concentration, emotions, sleep and general well-being. In addition, there are usually symptoms of cold limbs, recurrent fevers, palpitations, coloured dreams and urinary frequency.

Post Viral Syndrome This is something which has been described in medical text-books for many years. Sir William Osler, the doyen of physicians in the early 20th Century advocated the administration of strychnine as a stimulant after an attack of influenza.

In essence, Post Viral Syndrome seems to be a milder, shorter acting version of ME.

Intestinal Candidiasis The potential of the thrush organism, *Candida albicans*, to displace the normal protective bacteria in the bowel could cause the condition of Chronic Fatigue. It is suggested if there are recurrent attacks of vaginal thrush, oral thrush, abdominal bloating, alternating diarrhoea in someone who has had repeated courses of steroids, long term acne treatment with antibiotics, or the oral contraceptive pill for several years.

IT IS VITAL TO SEEK A MEDICAL OPINION IF THERE IS ANY ALTERATION IN BOWEL HABIT.

Hypoglycaemia Low blood sugar following a meal can occur as a result of 'reactive hypoglycaemia.' It may be associated with intestinal candidiasis. It is suggested by mood swings around meal times, premenstrual syndrome, sugar craving and binge eating.

Depression This problem can cause absolute exhaustion. If there are suicidal features then medical help should be sought.

Multiple Food Allergies These can also occur in the presence of intestinal candidiasis. People with a history of asthma and eczema may also be prone to other allergic manifestations.

In addition to these, but of more importance are chronic respiratory, cardiac and bowel disorders, degenerative neurological disease and malignancies.

IT IS VITAL THAT A MEDICAL OPINION BE SOUGHT AND APPROPRIATE INVESTIGATIONS BE PERFORMED TO EXCLUDE ANY POTENTIALLY SERIOUS MEDICAL CONDITION.

The question of exercise

There is much debate as to whether it is better to push oneself through the fatigue state. Some people claim that absolute rest is essential, while others claim that the fatigue is 'all in the mind' so there is no rational reason to rest or avoid exercise. Still others suggest that gradually increasing 'graded' exercise is the answer. The problem with all of these pieces of advice is that they are treating all people as if they reacted the same way. This patently is not the case.

There are some people who will benefit from hard exercise, just as there are some who will be better avoiding exercise. This is one of the fundamental principles in homoeopathy. Treat the individual as an individual and tailor the treatment to the patient.

It might be useful to note the following principles

Better for exercise

Ignatia
Natrum muriaticum
Rhus toxicodendron
Sepia

Worse for exercise

Aconite
Alumina
Arnica
Arsenicum album
Bryonia
Calcarea carbonica
China officinalis
Gelsemium
Graphites
Iodum
Kali phos
Lycopodium
Mercurius solubilis
Natrum carbonicum
Natrum muriaticum (although may be better, as above)
Phosphoric acidum
Picric acidum
Zincum metallicum

As you can see, in fatigue states, the majority of types are worse for exertion. In my view this means that one should be wary of doing too much, too soon. Gentle graded exercise seems to suit most people, but it should ideally be increased under professional advice. There are relatively few types who do improve with the 'get out there and get active' approach.

HOMOEOPATHIC TREATMENT OF CHRONIC FATIGUE

In homoeopathy the diagnostic term is not as important as the individual's reaction to the particular problem. As we have seen in depression, for example, there are many remedies which might help, but which can only do so if they are appropriate for the individual. Their appropriateness is deduced by matching the remedy profile to the individual's symptom-profile.

The same applies in Chronic Fatigue. However, if exhaustion and Chronic Fatigue begin following a definite viral infection then two additional things might help. Firstly, the constitutional remedy may stimulate the body's natural recuperative forces (and some of the following remedies may be constitutional remedies). Secondly, a nosode, a sort of specific homoeopathic 'vaccine' to the viral illness can counter the after-effects of the said organism. The latter approach, however, needs to be given under the direction of a professional homoeopath.

Common emotions with Chronic Fatigue Syndrome are depression, anger and hostility (because the problems may be written off by many people as being 'psychological'), guilt and jealousy. If these are present it is certainly worth treating these also. (See appropriate chapters on these emotions.)

The following remedies have all been found beneficial in my own homoeopathic practice.

Alumina – for exhaustion, both physical and mental, in thin people who may seem to age prematurely. They are prone to muscular weakness and 'paralytic' states. They want everything doing quickly, which will annoy them because their weakness and exhaustion will not permit them to be quick. They tend to suffer from dryness of the skin and all the mucous membranes. They fear that they might go mad.

Ammonium carbonicum – for post viral type exhaustion in types who tend to suffer from repeated colds and respiratory infections. They tend to be slow and lethargic, suffer from asthma and be fairly stout. Women may tend to have heavy periods. When ill they dislike water, never bathe, so they tend to lounge around and 'fester.' They hate stormy weather which increases their gloominess.

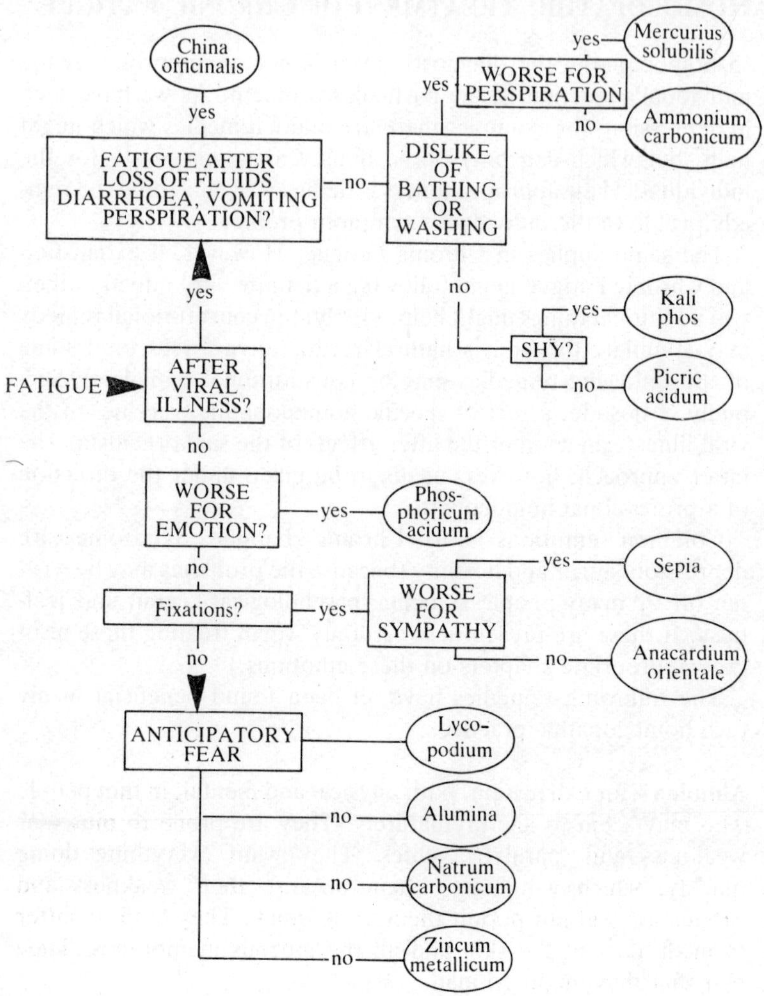

EXHAUSTION AND CHRONIC·FATIGUE

Anacardium orientale – one of the classical remedies for nervous exhaustion. There are quite fixed ideas, feelings of being unreal, like an observer of one's own life. There is weakness of all the senses, great exhaustion and an irresistible urge to swear. This may be completely out of character. There is over-sensitivity and vindictiveness.

Calcarea carbonica – for melancholic, slow, congested types who have a tendency to be lethargic. They have many fears, dislike the open air and are prone to perspiring on the head and chest. Very useful if it is the constitutional remedy.

China officinalis – for exhaustion after an illness which has caused a loss of body fluids, eg, diarrhoea and vomiting, profuse perspiration, or blood loss. There is a tendency to suffer from headaches with an exquisitely tender scalp. They become apathetic, irritable with a tendency to want to offend other people. There is insomnia and there is weepiness.

Kali phos – a traditional remedy for the after-effects of influenza and influenza-like illnesses. There is marked fear, irritability and a tendency to be startled. There is aversion to social chat. Exhaustion is extreme. Dizziness is common and there may be a tendency to fall. They dislike being left alone. They are worse for exertion.

Lycopodium – for exhaustion in professional types who tend to worry in anticipation of events and engagements, although they usually perform well when the time comes. They may be prone to digestive problems. Can be quite irritable. May be very useful if it is the constitutional remedy.

Mercurius solubilus – for exhaustion in people who feel awful when they perspire during illness. They hate exertion because of the way they feel when they perspire. They feel depressed, weak and are prone to tremors and shaking. They may form pus easily, so that sore throats always produce exudate and bad breath, cuts tend to fester and they may suffer from body odour. Their tongue often shows the imprint of their teeth.

Natrum carbonica – for exhaustion in pale, stout, people who are very sensitive to all sorts of things, be it noise, chatter, music, thunderstorms and 'atmospheres.' They tend to be critical individuals who can develop dislikes of people for no very obvious reason. They are very apprehensive about performing any mental or physical exertion when they are ill.

Phosphoric acidum – for exhaustion in mild types who become indifferent to people, events and things about them. They feel weak when talking. Headaches are common, which are worse for noise. They are worse for mental exertion and study.

Picric acidum – for exhaustion and weakness of all muscles. There is complete apathy for everything, even the effort of talking. Any mental exertion seems to bring on a headache. There is no anxiety about the illness, however. There is no appetite and there is a curious sensation of the ground coming up to meet the individual.

Sepia – for melancholic, weepy types who do not like sympathy, yet who dislike being left alone. They feel faint and weak, especially in the mornings. They can become very depressed and do not want to do anything. However, if they can be encouraged to take up some favourite activity, eg, dancing, they may seem to 'come alive.'

Zincum metallicum – for extreme exhaustion, fatigue and low spirits in tremulous, restless types who think slowly. Indeed, so slow do the thought processes seem, that the individual tends to repeat questions to buy time to answer. There is over-sensitivity and irritability over minor things. The memory is poor. Often there is a metallic taste in the mouth.

CHAPTER 14

Sleep Problems

Blessings on him who invented sleep,
the mantle that covers all human thoughts.
Miguel de Cervantes, *Don Quixote*

To such a madcap as the worthy Don Quixote the mantle of sleep must indeed have seemed a welcome night-garment. Unfortunately, for up to 40 per cent of the population at some time, and 10 per cent regularly, sleep can be an elusive butterfly.

Normal sleep and insomnia

Research in sleep laboratories has shown that during uninterrupted sleep a young adult drifts through four progressively deeper stages of non-rapid eye movement sleep (NREM sleep), associated with slow wave activity on the electroencephalogram (EEG or brain wave tracing). After about ninety minutes the first episode of rapid eye movement sleep (REM sleep) is entered, when muscle relaxation takes place and dreaming occurs. These REM episodes recur about five times during a sleep of 7–8 hours and occupy about 25 per cent of the total.

However, sleep time is not to be equated with 'good sleep.' While some people awake refreshed after only four or five hours sleep, some people will not be satisfied unless they have had their 'full eight hours' of unbroken sleep. Insomnia is therefore a subjective complaint.

A reasonable working definition of insomnia could therefore be 'a complaint of difficulty in initiating and/or maintaining sleep which is satisfying.'

Some causes of insomnia

It is a fact that the pattern of sleep varies with age. The amount of 'slow wave' sleep is reduced so that periods of wakefulness increase to cause broken, fragmented and unsatisfying sleep. To compensate for this many people take to having cat-naps, which of course will reduce the need for night-time sleep.

The expectation of sleep is often part of the problem, since people expect to need and get eight hours. The reality, however, is that as one gets into middle and later life the sleep requirement falls to about six hours. Consequently, as long as one does not feel tired upon waking there is no need for more. The tendency to take cat-naps, therefore, will only rob you of sleep during the night.

Apart from the normal changes that take place in the sleep cycle with age, most cases of correctable insomnia can be attributed to depression, anxiety, pain and drugs.

It obviously makes no sense to treat insomnia caused by painful conditions with sedatives or hypnotic medications. Similarly, emotional problems are merely numbed by the use of sleeping pills. And finally, if a drug has sleep disturbance as a side effect, it is clearly an unacceptable drug.

Caffeine in tea and coffee, various breathing tablets, diuretics, anti-depressants and Beta-blockers can all cause insomnia. Indeed, paradoxically so can many hypnotics themselves. The problem is that they tend to reduce REM sleep, thereby eventually causing wakefulness as tolerance increases to the drug.

Self-help measures

It is important that you do not make any alteration in your orthodox medication without first consulting your doctor.

Stop drinking tea or coffee after tea-time is worth doing, possibly going onto a herbal tea such as chamomile, peppermint, sage or rose-hip. Herbal tea-bags of all of these are available from most health shops. I find that they are best taken fairly weak, any bitterness being countered by about quarter of an inch worth of cut liquorice root, or a half spoonful of honey.

It is important not to overload the stomach last thing at night. A small snack is acceptable, although cheese and chocolate may keep you awake.

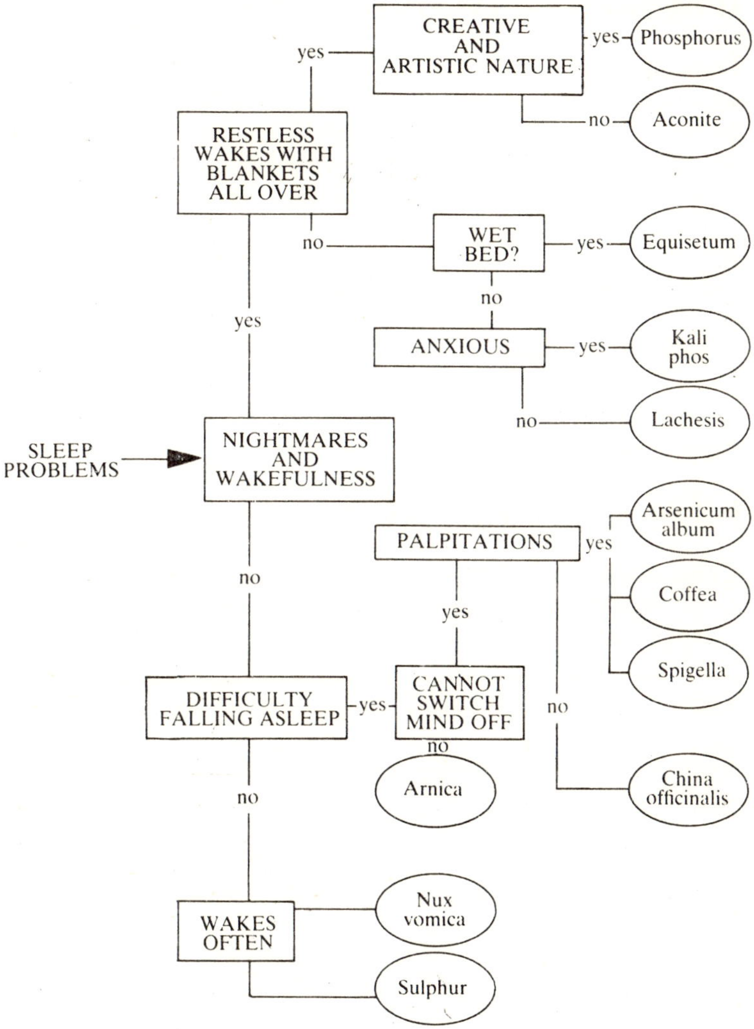

SLEEP PROBLEMS

Smoking last thing at night might make you feel relaxed, but it will in fact heighten your wakefulness and delay sleep.

Finally while alcohol is fairly good at inducing sleep, it may well cause broken sleep by reason of its diuretic effect. A little may be useful, but too much is likely to be too much.

Homoeopathic Treatment of Sleep Problems

From the above discussion it should be clear that if there is a significant emotional problem which is disturbing sleep, it should be the main target of treatment. Thus, the chapters on sadness and depression, and fear are worth consulting again.

The following remedies might also be of use.

Aconite – if there is a tendency to wake from a nightmare with the blankets all over the place after a restless period.

Arnica – feels exhausted, but unable to sleep. The bed feels hard.

Arsenicum album – for restlessness and anxiety. Wakes in the early hours. May have periodic upsets in sleep.

Belladonna – if the legs are restless and jerk you awake.

China officinalis – if thoughts crowd in at night. Especially if debilitated from diarrhoea, excess perspiration, blood loss, excessive laxative usage.

Coffea – if unable to switch off. Starts awake at the slightest noise.

Equisetum – for nightmares, especially if there is a bed-wetting tendency in a child.

Ignatia – if there is an unstoppable yearning to yawn repeatedly. Sleep won't come. Tend to be changeable, hysterical types.

Kali phosphoricum – for anxious types who suffer from recurrent nightmares and night terrors when under pressure.

Lachesis – for nightmares in jealous, talkative types who tend to get bloated. Often suffer from Premenstrual Syndrome, when the nightmares may be more frequent.

Nux Vomica – if there is indigestion after too rich food. May wake in a bad mood.

Phosphorus – if there are nightmares in creative, artistic types.

Spigelia – if kept awake by palpitations every night.

Sulphur – if tends to talk, grunt, snore in fitful sleep. Tends to stick the limbs outside the bed because they feel hot.

CHAPTER 15

Body Image and Eating Disorders

O wad some Pow'r the giftie gie us
To see oursels as others see us!
It wad frae mony a blunder free us,
And foolish notion.

Robert Burns

Imagery is important to all thinking creatures. We recognise people, animals and objects by the established image which we have of them. This conceptualisation about what things are, is not restricted to the sense of vision. Indeed, to someone who has been blind all their life there is no 'visual' image of, for example, a cow. Their conception of the cow is more likely to be built up from the senses of touch, hearing and smell. Clearly, giving a blind child a toy model of a cow in order to teach them about the cow is likely to lead to a false image of the animal which in reality is large, hairy and possibly smelly.

Apart from having images of the outside world it is important for us to have images of ourselves. It is part of knowing about one's individuality.

The image of oneself may not accord with the way that others see us. And indeed, other people probably have a more accurate physical image of you than you have yourself, because you can only see yourself in a mirror, while others can see you in 3-Dimensions.

The image which we present to the world, our persona, is the product of many things. It is partly geared by our physical body and attributes, our mental state and our emotional mix. It is not entirely a conscious projection, although we may often do much to alter our 'image,' to make ourselves look more assertive, more academic, more attractive, or whatever. Depending on all of these sorts of things we may project an image ranging from the fiercest of tigers to the most introspective shrinking violet.

If all is well our self-esteem, which includes the image one has of one's own body, will run high. If there is a background disturbance, however, then the body image may become grossly impaired. This can cause a vicious circle, because the image can further reduce the self-esteem to heighten the emotional imbalance and cause further problems with the body image. This may lead to a fixed idea forming, resulting in a problem such as an eating disorder.

The dysmorphophobias

There are a recognised group of conditions called the dysmorphophobias, which are all characterised by an unhappiness about the image of the body. The term is derived from the Greek words, *dus*, meaning ill; *morphe*, meaning form; and *phobos*, meaning fear.

The image of the body becomes distorted so that the individual takes drastic action, either physically or mentally to alter the image. This can vary from self-mutilation and suicidal attempts to binge-eating or starvation.

Anorexia nervosa is the commonest and best known of these problems. Figures about its incidence vary immensely, depending upon criteria of diagnosis. It is thought to occur in about 1 per cent of adolescent girls and young women in their early 20s who become fixated about slimming and dieting. Some groups do seem to be particularly susceptible, however. For example, dance students have been found to have an incidence of 20 per cent.

Countless theories abound as to its nature. Some advocate a biochemical or physiological aberration causing a hormonal upset which robs the individual of their appetite. Others suggest that the whole problem is emotional, resulting from a fear of becoming fat, or of growing up. By starving, or regurgitating food the metabolism is certainly affected, so that the periods stop and weight is progressively lost.

THIS IS A DANGEROUS CONDITION, SO ANYONE WHO DEVOTES MUCH OF THEIR ENERGY AND ATTENTION TO DIETING AND SLIMMING SHOULD CONSULT A DOCTOR.

Bulimia, the other side of the coin, where the individual becomes obsessed with food may in fact occur in the same individual. It may be that the two represent poles of a fluctuating problem, related to eating and body image. With this problem there may be tastes for peculiar foods, which then have to be consumed in large quantities – binge eating – often to the extent that the individual has to be sick before starting to eat again. Indeed, during a binge, the calorific intake can increase to five times the daily requirement. At its extreme, people have been known to take in twenty-five times their normal intake!

Most people with this problem have a cycle of binging and purging, in which an enormous intake is followed by a feeling that they need to 'purge' the system. This may involve self-induced vomiting, the taking of laxatives, diuretics, or a punishing regime of hard exercise.

The incidence of bulimia is not known. It seems to occur in a slightly older age group (20–25 years) than anorexia. It is thought that up to 5 per cent of this age group have a real problem, while between 20 and 30 per cent binge and purge themselves occasionally.

BINGE-EATING CAN RAPIDLY GET OUT OF CONTROL AND CAN BECOME DANGEROUS, SO ANYONE TEMPTED TO BINGE-EAT SHOULD CONSULT A DOCTOR.

Homoeopathic Treatment of Body Image Problems and Eating Disorders

As mentioned above, it is always sensible to consult a doctor first. Homoeopathy can help, but it should be used in consultation with a doctor.

There are many possible reasons why people do develop body image problems which result in eating disorders. If a dominant emotion comes to the surface then this should be the target of treatment. Of course, if the constitutional remedy is known then this will always help.

In order to simplify matters I have divided the remedies which I have found of use into two groups.

Anorexia

I use the term here, not in its strict psychiatric sense, but for those cases where there is an aversion to food and a fixation about the body image – which the individual feels to be too obese.

Alumina – while this is generally considered a useful remedy in middle and later life, there are many young women in their late teens and twenties who are susceptible to the actions of this remedy. They tend to be very thin to begin with and have a slight tremor at rest. They lose their appetite completely and fear obesity. The food they do like is unusual, eg, the crusts of bread, the rind of bacon, the pith of fruit.

Aurum metallicum – for loss of appetite and dislike of one's own body in melancholic types who may contemplate suicide. Their gradual starvation of themselves may be such a 'painless' death-wish!

Causticum – for loss of appetite in those types who are sympathetic to the needs of others. They may sympathise with others who have a weight problem and unconsciously go on a slimming diet. If they think about their own problems they feel worse, so they focus on others and their own dieting which becomes a fixed idea. Useful for those people who develop a problem which started after trying to help a friend or relative.

Natrum muriaticum – where there is loss of appetite, except for salt and salty foods in melancholic types who are worse for sympathy and consolation. They may develop fixed ideas about becoming fat and become obsessed with slimming and dieting.

Picric acidum – for loss of appetite and general exhaustion in types who are worse post-virally. (See last chapter.) They are worse for mental exertion.

Thuja occidentalis – for complete loss of appetite and fixed ideas about the body image. Generally very thin with a tendency to develop warts. Always feel hurried.

BULIMIA

Once again, this is not used in the strict psychiatric sense, but for those cases where there is a ravenous appetite, a desire to binge and a fear of starving.

Ammonium carbonicum – where there is a huge appetite that is quickly satiated, but which develops rapidly again. There is a general aversion to washing and water, so that the individual may neglect body hygiene and develop body odour.

Argentum nitricum – when there is a desire to binge on chocolate and sweet foods in someone prone to fears and anticipatory anxiety.

Calcarea carbonica – for ravenous appetite in slow, melancholic types with a tendency to constipation. Their motivation is usually a genuine fear that they might starve if they don't keep eating.

China officinalis – for ravenous appetite in people who have had a recent infectious illness associated with loss of body fluids. The state is likely to be temporary, although some cases do persist and develop a real eating disorder. There is a tendency to want to emotionally 'hurt' people.

Graphites – for ravenous appetite in melancholic women with a tendency towards obesity. Seafood, however, may make them feel quite ill, even if they have craved it.

Iodum – where there is ravenous appetite, but still a problem in putting weight on.

Phosphorus – for increased appetite in artistic, creative types who may even feel themselves to be clairvoyant. They may binge to the point of vomiting upon sweet or salty foods.

Pulsatilla – for increased appetite in plump, fair-haired types who are changeable emotionally, better for being outdoors and who weep easily. They like sympathy. They generally hate fatty foods but may binge on 'healthy' foods like salads. Generally, they are quite thirstless.

Sabadilla – for increased appetite in timid, shy types. They develop curious ideas about themselves and about their bodies. They may imagine that they have some disease which can only be kept in check by constant eating and continued 'nourishment' of the tissues.

Sulphur – for increased appetite in dominant, 'ragged philosopher' types who tend to lean, slouch and fidget. They binge because they have a fear of starvation.

Zincum metallicum – for ravenous appetite in the late morning.

CHAPTER 16

Premenstrual Syndrome & The Menopause

The premenstrual syndrome (PMS), like fear, has three components – emotional, physical and behavioural. Usually the problems start from the middle of the menstrual cycle and continue until the period has finished.

Most women experience some premenstrual symptoms at some stage. For 30–40 per cent these symptoms can be so troublesome that they are forced to seek medical aid. About 5 per cent find their symptoms so bad that they are unable to function effectively in their daily lives.

The medical literature cites over 150 symptoms which have been attributed to PMS. The commonest are:-

Emotional Depression, anxiety, irritability, hostility, jealousy, weepiness, indifference.

Physical Bloating of the abdomen, bloating of the breasts, bloating of the neck, headache, fluid retention, acne.

Behavioural Aggression, avoidance of others, altered sex drive and pattern.

Uncertain causes

Although there are many theories concerning the underlying cause of PMS, none have been proven. In the past a purely psychological cause was postulated, it being suggested that women who suffered from it had a high 'neuroticism' level. Thankfully, this antiquated and blinkered view is gradually disappearing.

The study of twins has suggested that a genetic factor could be involved. It has been found that the incidence of PMS is higher in identical twins (who develop from the same egg and therefore have identical genetic information) than in non-identical twins (who develop from two eggs, so are absolute individuals with different genetic information).

Since the symptoms start in the second half of the menstrual cycle it seems logical to assume that ovulation and the hormonal balance in the second half of the cycle have something to do with PMS. Let us, therefore, consider the hormones responsible for the menstrual cycle.

To begin with it is important to appreciate that the output of hormones affecting the reproductive system in women, is governed by a feedback loop. This involves the hypothalamus and the pituitary gland, which are both found in the brain. The ovaries, which produce the eggs, form the second part of the loop.

The ovaries have a finite number of eggs which can become fertilised throughout a woman's reproductive life. Before fertilisation can occur, however, an egg has to be primed, developed and transported from the ovary towards the womb via one of the Fallopian Tubes. Under the influence of the female hormones the egg is primed and developed up to the point of 'ovulation', when it is released to begin its journey towards the womb.

The pituitary gland starts the cycle off when the circulating blood level of *oestrogen* and *progesterone* (the ovarian hormones) falls below a certain level after the period has finished. This causes the release of *Follicle Stimulating Hormone* (FSH), *Luteinising Hormone* (LH) and *Prolactin*. These hormones have an effect on ovarian function.

FSH causes a Graffian Follicle, containing the potential egg to become primed. As it develops, the Follicle starts to secrete oestrogen. This first half of the cycle is known as the *Follicular phase*. During it, the endometrium of the womb begins to build up in thickness.

The oestrogen level builds up to a peak at mid-cycle, when LH starts to take over to help stimulate 'ovulation'. The second half of the cycle, when the egg is transported towards the womb, is associated with further development of the egg and increased build up of the endometrium of the womb, in readiness for implantation of the egg if it becomes fertilised. This half sees a rise in the level of progesterone from the *Corpus Luteum or yellow body* (a structure which develops from the ruptured Graffian Follicle after the release of the egg) as a result of stimulation from LH and Prolactin. This is called the *Luteal Phase*.

At this point either a fertilised egg becomes implanted or the hormone levels fall, causing the shedding of the endometrial layer with the bleeding of the menstrual period.

The role of oestrogen is to develop and maintain the reproductive tract and the female sex organs. It has an effect upon the metabolism of bones (a lack at the menopause causing osteoporosis), upon the mineral and fluid balance of the body, upon the mucous membranes and the skin. The peak level of oestrogen occurs in mid-cycle with ovulation, although there is a smaller peak later in the Luteal Phase.

The role of progesterone is to nurture the tissues in readiness for the reception of a fertilised egg. It also has an effect upon the muscles and ligaments of the body. Some of its action may affect the musculature of the bowel. It also has an effect on the skin, an excess sometimes producing acne. The peak level of progesterone occurs in the middle of the Luteal Phase.

A simplified view of the hormonal changes in the menstrual cycle is shown on page 143. A glance at the levels of hormones will make it clear that there is great scope for an 'imbalance' to occur between oestrogen and progesterone. And from what has already been said, there are ways in which either hormone could account for some of the symptoms of PMS. For example, a relative oestrogen excess could account for bloating and fluid retention. Similarly, a relative progesterone excess could cause bowel cramps, backache, fatigue and acne.

Because some symptoms seem to fit with one hormone rather than the other, the artificial model is sometimes used of the *oestrogenic* or the *progestogenic* woman. The oestrogenic type is thought of as tending to be stouter, more troubled with bloating and having fairly heavy periods. By contrast, the progestogenic woman is thought of as being slimmer, more troubled with spasm pains, even though the periods are lighter, and with a tendency to develop acne.

This model is quite attractive, except that in practice it becomes quite obviously too restrictive. There are numerous overlaps in

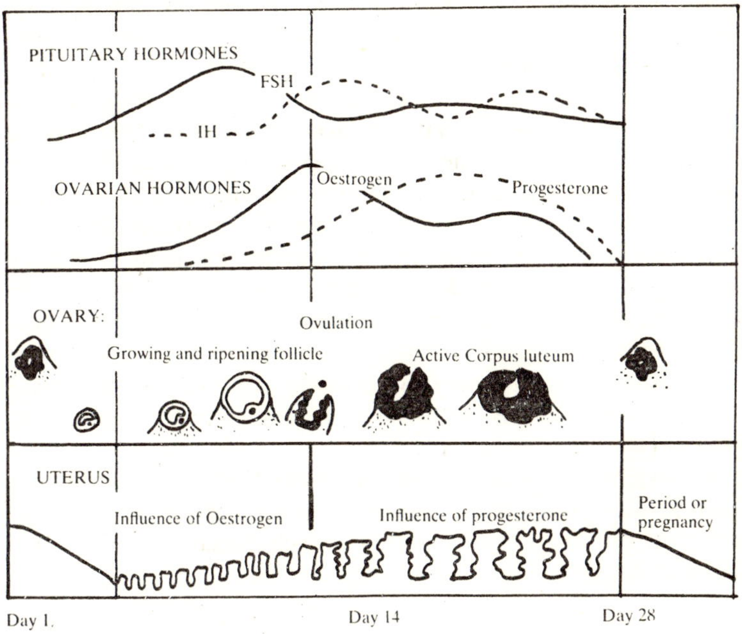

THE HORMONAL, OVARIAN AND ENDOMETRIAL CHANGES OF THE MENSTRUAL CYCLE

symptoms, as well as many symptoms which clearly cannot be accounted for on the basis of hormonal physiology.

There are equally good theories about the role of kidney produced hormonal agents, neurotransmitters and the body's endorphin levels. None account for all of the possible symptoms and, as I stated earlier, none have been proven.

Imbalances in other parts of the body metabolism may also be involved as secondary effects. For example, it may be that glucose control becomes imperfect, either because the circulating hormones interfere with insulin action, or because of some effect on appetite or eating which then affects the glucose level. Whichever is the case, it does seem that some women benefit from taking smaller meals more frequently. Indeed, eating carbohydrate or starch foods every 3 hours (although not increasing the overall daily calorie intake) often brings about an improvement in symptoms. This may be because hypoglycaemia (low blood glucose) can cause quite marked mood swings in people.

Another possible factor is the development of a relative deficiency of Pyridoxine (Vitamin B_6), caused by the high level of circulating oestrogen. The low Pyridoxine level could then have an affect on various neurotransmitters, causing some of the mood swings, the fatigueability and the cramps. Treatment should be restricted to 50–100 milligrams per day for no more than three months at a time. High doses above 2 grams per day (ie, twenty times the above dose) can produce significant nerve damage. There is also some evidence that prolonged dosage (more than 6 months) can result in a neuropathy (a condition affecting various nerves of the body) which is, fortunately, reversible upon stopping the treatment.

Finally, there is a quite a lot of evidence that some women drop their levels of fatty acids. This seems to account for the beneficial effect of *Oil of Evening Primrose*, which contains the fatty acid *Gamolenic Acid*.

Homoeopathic Treatment of PMS

From the above discussion it should be clear that PMS is an extremely complicated tapestry. While many of the theories seem to explain some of the features, none come anywhere near explaining all. And this is, of course, inevitable. The problem is that it is another blanket term describing several different conditions, the linking feature being that they affect women in the second half of their menstrual cycle. The fact that over 150 symptoms have been attributed to it implies that there are many different reactions to the underlying condition.

This is yet again where the homoeopathic approach has much to offer. Rather than trying to explain the underlying pathology, the aim is to delineate symptom-profiles from the multiplicity of symptoms which have been described. The correct match of remedy to person will usually bring about swift relief over one cycle, and hopefully clear it after three treatments.

It has to be noted, however, that some women will improve in various aspects of their PMS, but change their pattern to become more like another remedy-profile. If this happens then the new remedy should be used, probably with good effect.

Taking the Remedy for PMS

My own method of prescribing for PMS is to give 2 tablets of the 30C potency, three times a day for the first three days after the period has stopped. This should be repeated after the following two cycles, making three treatments in total. (Also see *Notes on Taking the Remedies* at the start of Part 3.)

The Major Remedies

In my experience the following four remedies will deal with the reaction patterns of about 75 per cent of PMS sufferers.

Lachesis

This remedy is derived from a snake venom and as such it explains many of the symptoms of this pattern of PMS.

Emotional features There is suspiciousness, jealousy, talkativeness, irritability and anger.

The suspicions can be self-destroying. It can be a suspicion about the neighbours, about people talking about her, or about her husband's fidelity.

The jealousy becomes acute and can be directed at anyone in the family. There can be jealousy of another's ability, health, willpower – anything.

There may be a reputation for being a chatterbox. Certainly there is no holding back during the premenstrual phase. She will often talk openly about problems, suspicions etc.

Irritability is acute and can be violent. There is a desire to hurt with words. It is not just a matter of sticking the knife in, there is a desire to twist it as well. This gives the impression of the Jeykyl and Hyde change in personality. The PMS personality is always the ill tempered Hyde.

Concentration goes and there is likely to be weepiness.

Physical features There is a sensation of bloating. The abdomen, breasts and neck may all be affected, so that she doesn't like to wear a belt, bra or high neck-line or scarf.

There may be fluid retention. Indeed, a gain of 2kg is not unusual during the premenstrual phase.

There may be skin problems, most of which will have a faint blue or purplish tinge.

There may be a hammering headache.

Most physical symptoms start on the left side.

All pains are better once the period starts.

Behavioural features There may be physical aggression. There may be a tendency to throw things.

The sex drive is enhanced during the period itself.

Lilium tigrinum

This remedy is similar to Sepia, but is often described as a 'hot Sepia.' (See later.)

Emotional features There is profound depression, weepiness most of the time for minor or no reason, fears of having serious illness, a need to hurry and a fiery temper.

The depression is quite severe, more marked than in the Sepia with which it compares. Tears will come often for no obvious reason. In the middle of a conversation she may suddenly burst out crying.

Fears of cancer or other serious illness are always heightened premenstrually.

There is a constant pressure to keep going, keep moving, albeit without any definite aim. It is rather like running fast to keep still.

The temper is different from the Lachesis. In Lilium tigrinum there is irritability, but the outbursts of anger are merely an extension of that. There is no desire to emotionally hurt or wound the target of the anger. There is more likely to be a tendency to swear.

They hate sympathy and consolation and may be bad-tempered about it, even although they like to be the centre of attention.

They cannot be pleased.

Physical features There are many symptoms related to the pelvis. There is a dragging-down sensation in the vagina and the rectum.

It can be so bad that there is a need to sit and cross the legs for fear that the womb may actually fall out.

There is always a feeling of heat. There is a sensation that one may faint because they are too hot, or because the room is too warm.

There may be the need to go urgently to open the bowels, the motions always feeling hot.

There may be a need to pass urine frequently. Again, it will probably feel hot, as if they have 'cystitis.'

Behavioural features They are better for getting out and walking in the open air.

The sex drive is very markedly enhanced during the premenstrual phase.

Natrum muriaticum

Salt is the common name for this remedy, which might be guessed from some of it features.

Emotional features There is depression, weakness and lethargy, irritability and weepiness when on their own.

There is a background melancholy which is exacerbated in the premenstrual phase. They do not like to talk about it, unlike Lachesis.

They feel drained as the premenstrual period advances, as if they become progressively drained of salt and energy. At the end of the day they flop.

Their irritability is marked. They may fly into a temper at trifles. The thing to appreciate is that they will always be like this, the premenstrual phase perhaps merely increasing the frequency of the outbursts.

They have no sense of humour and hate having jokes played on them.

They feel weepy, but will not let the tears come until they are on their own.

They hate sympathy and consolation, but unlike Lilium tigrinum they will not rage. Rather will they want to go off and cry on their own.

Physical features They are cold, whereas Lilium Tigrinum is always hot.

They are always thirsty and they crave salt or salty foods.

They may suffer from hammering headaches preceded by zig-zag vision.

They often get palpitations.

They suffer from skin problems, eg eczema, acne, cold sores. They also tend to get hang-nails on their fingers.

Their periods tend to be less regular than the other remedies mentioned.

They may get pains after passing urine.

Behavioural features They want to be on their own to weep or mull things over. They still like people in the house.

They dislike exercise.

Their sex drive disappears. They may avoid sex because it can be painful, a result of not having much vaginal lubrication.

Sepia

This remedy is prepared from the inky juice of the cuttlefish. Think of it as a vulnerable type remedy with a protective shell of indifference.

Emotional features There is depression, indifference, lethargy, over-sensitivity, irritability and weepiness.

The depression is, as with Natrum muriaticum, a background feature. It is merely heightened premenstrually.

Indifference is the characteristic feature, however. There is a loss of interest in the well-being of relatives, partners and friends. When they are feeling really bad they can be totally indifferent to the plight of their closest loves.

The indifference can produce total lethargy and apathy. There is a feeling that nothing is worth doing.

They are very sensitive to criticism and are easily offended.

Their irritability is not so marked as either Lachesis or Lilium tigrinum. It is shorter lived.

They will weep when talking about their symptoms, but they dislike sympathy or consolation. Their reaction is to be bad-tempered, although not as marked as Lilium tigrinum.

They hate being on their own, although like to have room to themselves.

Physical features They are cold, unlike Lilium tigrinum.

They get a dragging down sensation in the pelvis, although not as marked as in Lilium tigrinum.

There is often a feeling of having 'a ball' inside them. If there is a stomach problem, they get a solid feeling like a ball inside the abdomen. Similarly, they can experience this in the rectum or in the pelvis.

Headaches are common at the back of the head.

Behavioural features There is a desire to be left alone, albeit with someone else in the house.

They are better if they can be persuaded to do some exercise.

There is a complete aversion to sex.

The Minor Remedies

The following remedies will usually deal with those cases not helped by the major remedies.

Calcarea carbonica – for PMS where breast tenderness, slowness and congestion in the pelvis is common.

Causticum – for PMS where there is irritability, great pessimism about the future. Thinking about their problems makes them much worse.

Graphites – for PMS where there is constipation, gross fluid retention and a flare-up of skin troubles.

Nux vomica – for PMS in high-achievers who tend to use stimulants. They are extremely fiery and will argue about everything.

Pulsatilla – for PMS in generally shy, timid types. They suffer from wildly changeable symptoms, often of a quite unusual nature. For example, they may get a headache which is better for having a very hot shower.

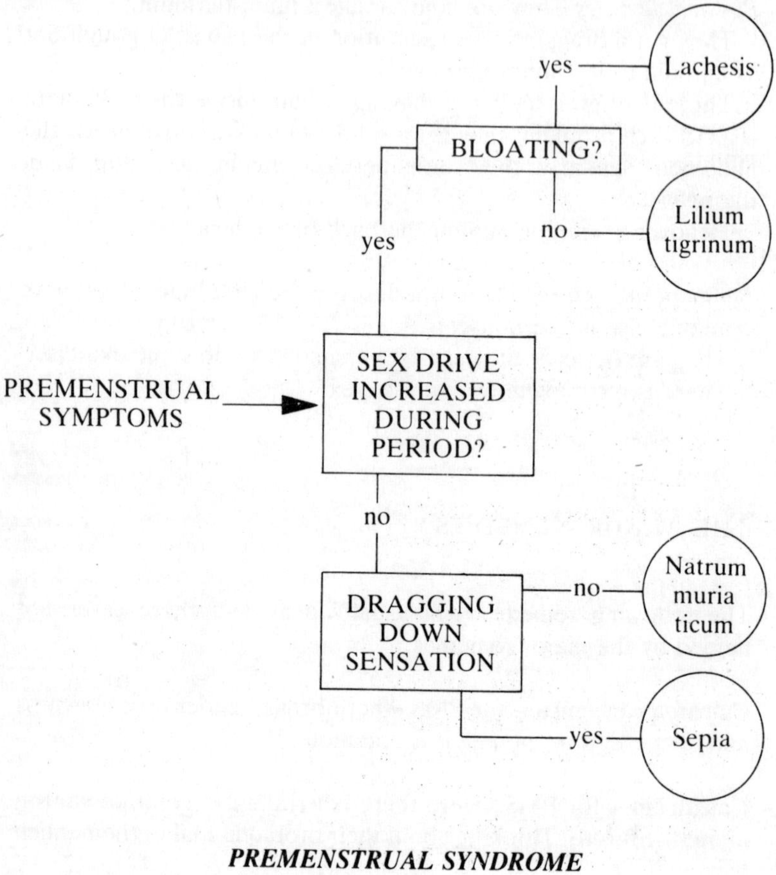

PREMENSTRUAL SYNDROME

THE MENOPAUSE

The menopause can be a traumatic time for many women. It marks the cessation of the reproductive part of their lives, so it is a time of great change. There are alterations in the hormone levels as the ovaries stop producing eggs, there is a loss of bone substance (which may produce osteoporosis) and there is a psychological adjustment to be made.

The main culprit in this time of change seems to be the hormone 'oestrogen.' As it falls during the menopause it causes menopausal flushing, vaginal dryness and soreness. There is also a complicated relationship with the metabolism of calcium and other minerals which may result in bone loss and osteoporosis.

Understandably, because of the great changes taking place in the individual's life, it is also a time when body image and self-esteem become distorted. Post-menopausal depression is, therefore, extremely common.

Hormone Replacement Therapy (HRT) is now widely advocated as women approach and pass through the menopause, in order to minimise problems like flushing and vaginal soreness, and to prevent osteoporosis. Not everyone can tolerate this treatment, however, and indeed not everyone chooses to have it.

There are things that individual women can do to minimise problems in both their menopause and their post-menopausal years.

Stop Smoking

It really is never too late to stop. Although the mechanism has not been fully delineated, there is no doubt that cigarette smoking is a major risk factor for heart disease, all cancers and osteoporosis.

Exercise

Moderate exercise seems to be more beneficial than strenuous exercise. Listen to your body and do not attempt any exercise beyond your limits. Remember the decades. What is reasonable for an average 40 year old would be quite strenuous for an average 50 year old and so on. For example, a fit fifty year old woman could still be playing badminton twice a week, swimming and golfing. A fit 70 year old could play a round of golf a week, swim or take a brisk walk, while for an 80 year old a walk twice a week would be fine. If in doubt about your limits have a chat with your doctor.

DIET

There are two main factors to boost in your diet:

Calcium
Phyto-oestrogens (plant oestrogens)

Calcium A recent conference in Copenhagen advised that women at the menopause should take in 1,000–1,500 mg of calcium daily. Once through it into the Third Age an intake of 800–1,000 mg would be adequate.

To give you some idea of the calcium content of foods, a pint of semi-skimmed milk contains about 650 mg; a 5oz pot of yoghurt contains 240 mg; and 1oz of Cheddar cheese contains about 200 mg.

It is important, however, not to exceed 1,500 mg daily after the menopause (unless of course advised to by your doctor) because of the potential risk of developing kidney stones.

Phyto-oestrogens It has been known since the 1970s that some crops used for animal pasture have oestrogenic activity. It is also known that some plants contain natural chemicals – 'phyto-oestrogens.'

In 1990 an Australian team looked at the effect of these naturally occurring plant oestrogens on women who had passed through the menopause. In order to do this the women had their diets supplemented with soya flour, various sprouts and a small amount of linseed oil. They found a very beneficial effect upon the cells of the vagina, compatible with improved oestrogen activity.

In this context 'sprouts' are various pulses and seeds which are moistened and allowed to sprout eg, soya beans and red clover.

In addition to the phyto-oestrogens, pulses are also good sources of protein, Vitamins B and C. They also have smaller amounts of iron, magnesium and calcium.

Adding soya to the diet instead of some of the red meat, plus some of the other sprouts, eg, lentils, two or three times a week may result in symptomatic improvement.

IT IS IMPORTANT THAT PULSES SHOULD ALWAYS BE COOKED TO DESTROY THE PHYTIC ACID AND TOXIC LECITHINS IN THEM, OTHERWISE THEY CAN PRODUCE A SEVERE GASTRO-ENTERITIS.

The remedies which I find most useful in the menopause are the following:

Aurum metallicum – if there are frequent hot flushes in melancholic types who may sink so low in their mood that they feel suicidal. They may be quite critical of others and have temper tantrums. They are worse for concentration.

Graphites – for lethargic depression at the menopause, when there is enhanced appetite. These individuals tend to be timid and indecisive. They tend to be very emotional and may cry at music.

Lachesis – if there are flushings, a bloated feeling and depression at the menopause in talkative, jealous, suspicious types. A classic remedy for post-menopausal depression.

Sepia – if there are flushes accompanied by a dragging down sensation in indifferent, lethargic types. They may be dragged out of themselves if they can be persuaded to do some favourite activity, eg, dancing.

Sulphur – if there is depression, perspiration and frequent flushing. They dislike being still, and tend to lean or slouch.

CHAPTER 17

Bad Habits

Sow an act, and you reap a habit.
Charles Reade (1814–1884)

All habits are a form of learned behaviour. We talk about some being good, in that they serve some useful purpose. On the other hand, we talk about bad habits when they are aesthetically unpleasant, hazardous to health or liable to lead to other problems.

Many habits start off fairly simply and seem quite innocuous. Parents of a thumb-sucking baby may initially regard the habit as a friend, in that it stops the crying, acts as a comfort and may even allow them some extra sleep. When it persists into late childhood or even into the teens, it is another matter. Trying to get the youngster to stop can then cause the greatest of problems.

The thing is that most of these habits become second nature. The individual may not appreciate that they are doing anything unusual. Attempting to stop proves difficult because a dependence is built up. Although it may not be obvious, there is always some gain involved in the habit.

In Chapter 5 we looked at various coping mechanisms. Well, habits are means of coping. From the child who sucks his thumb for comfort, to the adult with his alcohol and tobacco dependence, there is (initially at least) a lessening of tension. Removing that habit, that learned coping mechanism, causes a sudden surge of tension and an explosion in stress.

Unfortunately, when a weak coping mechanism like a habit has been in operation for a long time it induces stresses of its own.

The term 'breaking the habit' is not as simple as it is intended to sound. Rather than breaking the anchoring link with the individual, there is a risk of breaking the individual and leaving them to face a whole host of emotions until the healing process is complete.

Many people favour the 'cold turkey' approach, whereby the individual is suddenly deprived of their habit or addiction. The result is an unpleasant physical and psychological reaction. Others favour a graded reduction in the habit in order to allow the body to reduce its physical craving, minimise the extent of the physical withdrawal reaction, and maximise the confidence needed to finally lose the habit. In general, I favour the latter approach which seems the most logical. Having said that, there are some people who can only handle things if they throw themselves in at the deep end and 'get it over with quickly'. Again, it all reflects the individuality of people and their different needs.

HOMOEOPATHIC TREATMENT OF HABITS

As I mentioned above, I favour a graded reduction of the habit. Thus, in trying to stop some activity or another I usually advise a period of observation of how often the activity is done. This can be quite informative to the individual, because they may hardly be aware that they are doing anything out of the ordinary. For example, how many cigarettes are smoked on average, how many drinks are consumed, how often is the nose picked, how often are the nails bitten, how often is the hair twirled.

After the observation period comes the establishment of a realistic graded reduction program. Let us consider cigarette smoking as an example.

First, a definite 'stop smoking day' should be nominated and the daily intake be gradually reduced. The following way is my general method.

Start by dividing the day into three-hour periods – eg, 7am–10am, 10am–1pm, 1pm–4pm, 4pm–7pm, 7pm-bedtime.

The rationale for this is that only so many cigarettes are allowed per three hour period. It is not permitted to borrow one from another period, or to have one less in one period and an extra one at a later period. The whole idea is to induce some sense of discipline into the habit.

If a smoker is getting through 20 cigarettes a day, for example, then in the first week he ought to continue to smoke up to 20 cigarettes a day, but only permitting 4 in any of the three hour periods. If he decides only to have 3 in one period then that is good, he has already reduced his intake by 1 cigarette.

It is a good idea to have habit substitutes. In the case of cigarettes I advise cutting carrots and celery sticks to cigarette length and chewing them whenever a craving comes on. Liquorice roots are also good and can be conveniently carried around.

A help line is excellent help, if you can arrange to have people on the end of a telephone who won't mind you contacting them when you need a diversion (and this may be during the middle of the night!).

Finally, changing one's habitat is worth doing. By this I don't mean that one should move home, but that you should think of altering the places you go and the things you do which are generally associated with the habit. For example, stop going to the bar for a drink, avoid the canteen where everyone smokes, stop smoking out of doors, or only allow yourself to smoke in one place.

In addition, take up new interests. Do something outrageous. Choose something which you have never got around to, or which simply seems out of character. If you are changing your habits, you are changing yourself – start the way you mean to go on!

The reduction program should be done slowly, taking a long time if it is a long established habit. For example, the 20 a day cigarette smoker should do his reduction week by week. In week 1 he should allow himself 4 cigarettes in each three hour period, ie 20 a day. In week 2 he reduces by 1 cigarette per period, ie 15 a day. In week 3 he reduces by 1 cigarette per period, ie 10 a day. In week 4 he reduces by 1 cigarette per period, ie 5 a day. In week 5 he reduces to 2 cigarettes a day for three days, then 1 cigarette a day for three days, then on the last day he stops!

Such a reduction program has a good chance of success on its own, but it is important not to weaken. The supports are necessary and all help available should be taken until one has passed several months.

With addictive habits like tobacco and alcohol it is probably true to say that there is no safe time to test whether or not the habit is cured. One should assume it has, but tell oneself that there is no need to test it out, because it is no longer part of one's life.

Homoeopathic remedies do not provide an easy way for breaking a habit. They can help, if the indications are right. Their role is to reduce craving, rather than to stop the activity. It is, after all, the individual's willpower that is needed.

Taking the remedy for bad habits

It is important not to take the remedy for too long or too often. If it is the right one it will help.

My approach is to give 2 tablets of the 30C potency, three times a day for three days only at the start of the reduction program. This can be repeated just before the 'stopping day', or at about a month after the first treatment. It is worth repeating it for up to three days (less if there is no craving) a month after that. (See also the *Notes on Taking the Remedies* at the start of Part 3.)

Alcohol Dependence

The safe limit for alcohol is nowadays believed to be 21 units a week for a man and 14 units per week for a woman. A unit is taken as a measure of spirit, a glass of wine or a half pint of beer.

It is generally agreed that alcoholism or alcohol addiction is a dependency problem, characterised by both a physical and psychological dependence. The physical dependence means that unless the individual has their regular daily dosage, they experience symptoms and signs of withdrawal. These can be extremely unpleasant.

The psychological dependence usually starts first, because of the quick effect that alcohol has on relieving strain (a function of stress, remember). Missing the regular dose can cause the strain to become immediately apparent.

Men usually outnumber women by five to one. The figures given in the literature suggest that one in a hundred have a problem. However, most practitioners would consider this to be an underestimate.

Aconite – for the extreme anxiety and fear which occur if the daily dose is missed. A good remedy if the problem started after a severe trauma or shock.

Arsenicum album – for alcohol dependence in tidy, fussy types who take the alcohol to relieve their anxiety and restlessness. Useful for women who fall into the sherry bottle trap.

Lachesis – for alcohol dependence in talkative, suspicious, jealous types. They may tend to take bartenders and other bar customers into their confidence.

Nux vomica – for fiery high-achievers who tend to use all sorts of stimulants. They still suffer from over-use of alcohol, rich food and tobacco, developing a marked hangover effect.

Sulphur – for dominant, ragged philosopher types who tend to lean, lounge and slouch. They will drink anything and may be prone to binge-drinking.

Zincum metallicum – for nervous, tremulous types. They may drink to calm the nerves and the tremors, yet their stomachs may suffer from the alcohol.

When reducing alcohol consumption it is important to ensure a good vitamin intake. Plenty of fresh fruit and vegetables should be added to the diet.

Bed-Wetting

Bed-wetting, or nocturnal enuresis, is a common problem in childhood. It is the passage of urine during sleep. Often it can create an immense amount of tension in a whole household. The sufferer might be continually fearful of the parents' reaction, and other children in the home may suffer from the general air of irritability.

Bladder control develops slowly, the time needed being unique to the individual. It cannot be rushed.

Three out of four children will be dry by the age of three years, nine out of ten by the age of five, and probably less than five per cent will be troubled by the age of ten.

In the majority of children who have never been dry, bed-wetting is merely a delay in development – while development in all other areas remains normal. In less than five per cent bed-wetting is due to disease.

IF A CHILD HAS BEEN DRY FOR SOME TIME, THEN STARTS WETTING AGAIN, A MEDICAL OPINION SHOULD BE SOUGHT.

Countless treatments have been advocated over the years. The Ancient Egyptians used to give sufferers mouse pie at night. The Romans advised thrashing the inside of the legs with nettles. And in medieval times an ingenious alarm was devised, consisting of tying a toad between the knees. If the child passed urine the toad woke up – and immediately roused the child!

The important thing is to be understanding and consistent in your approach. This means that the child should not be made to feel guilty, by scolding, black-mailing, teasing or being threatened.

If the child has never been dry at night, then they should be told that the problem is not unusual and that it is not their fault. If they have started school then it will probably help to be told that there are possibly another three or four class-mates with the same problem.

One thing which should be discouraged is the bringing of the child into the parental bed after the wetting. If anything, this is liable to reinforce the problem.

The important thing is to break the vicious circle of tension, anxiety and embarrassment. By doing so, most children will be helped.

The following remedies may produce an effect swiftly.

Argentum nitricum – for bed-wetting in children who are fearful of all sorts of things. They are anxious about forthcoming events, sleep poorly and wet the bed.

Belladonna – for a tendency to bed-wet whenever there is an infection (not necessarily of the urinary system). There is restlessness during the night.

Equisetum – the classic remedy for childhood bed-wetting. Usually there is a vivid dream or a nightmare coincident with the bed-wetting.

Pulsatilla – for timid, shy, weepy children. They are changeable in nature and prefer being outdoors.

NAIL-BITING

This can be an almost intractable condition lasting almost throughout life in some people. They simply are not aware that they are doing it, yet are always envious of other people's beautifully manicured nails. When they are tense they will nibble more frequently, often causing bleeding.

There are many paints and varnishes on the market which sometimes work. However, even an unpleasant taste may not stop the addicted nail-biter. My usual advice is to look at the nails which are usually bitten most, then tape up completely the nails on both hands which are bitten least of all. Usually these are the little finger and the ring finger. The individual is then permitted to nibble to their heart's content on the remaining exposed nails. Each evening the taped nails are looked at, then immediately retaped. After two to three weeks the tapes are removed completely and one or two of the other nails are taped instead. This allows the individual to see how pleasant it is to have a grown, unbitten nail!

Obviously, the only nails they are allowed to bite are the exposed ones which have never been taped. Finally, after another two or three weeks the remaining nails are taped, so that the nail-biting has to stop. At the end of the last period, hopefully, there will be an end to the problem.

I have found the following remedies useful.

Ammonium bromatum – for an irritating, itchiness around the fingertips and under the nails, only relieved by biting the nails.

Argentum nitricum – for people who suffer from anticipatory fear. When they are very tense they tend to get diarrhoea. They often crave chocolate and bite their nails.

Arum triphyllum – when there is a tendency to bite and pick at the nails until they bleed.

Nose-Picking

This must rank as one of the most unpleasant of habits. Because of this, it is well worth trying to curb it with homoeopathic remedies.

Its onset is usually in childhood and may persist throughout life.

Arum triphyllum – when there is much crusting of the nose. The individual picks at the crusts until bleeding occurs.

Cina – for itching and picking of the nose in irritable, never satisfied types. May also grind teeth while asleep.

Natrum carbonicum – when there is a feeling of release from tension after 'boring' into the nose.

Sulphur – for nose-picking in dominant, lazy types who always fidget.

Thumb-Sucking

Here there may be a tendency to suck either the thumb or a favourite digit. The vast majority of thumb-suckers stop spontaneously before the age of ten.

Arsenicum album – in neat, tidy and fussy individuals. It might seem out of character with their overall neatness.

Phosphorus – for thumb-sucking in artistic people. The thumb might seem itchy or hot, but be relieved by sucking.

Pulsatilla – for thumb-sucking in gentle, timid types who are better for being outdoors.

Sulphur – in dominant types who tend to fidget. They may manage to curb the habit, yet sleep with the thumb in the mouth well into adulthood.

Tobacco Addiction

The greatest preventable threat to health is cigarette smoking. It can cause virtually any type of cancer, ischaemic heart disease, strokes and chronic respiratory disease. I thoroughly recommend the graded reduction method outlined earlier in this chapter.

There are no homoeopathic remedies which stop the individual from smoking, but the craving might be helped by the following.

Arsenicum album – for smoking in tidy, fussy, restless types who dislike the habit because of its messiness. They are very irritable when it is mentioned, however.

Ignatia – for smoking in hysterical types who make a big thing about their attempts to stop. They let everyone know how difficult it is for them.

Nux vomica – for fiery types who tend to use most stimulants. They say they actually like to smoke, yet dislike the constant bad taste they have, as well as the unpleasant 'thick head' in the morning.

Sulphur – for dominant types who tend to fidget and slouch. While they may be able to give up quite easily if they set their mind to it, they miss the fiddling with their hands.

Tranquilliser Dependence

In the 1960s, barbiturates and amphetamines were the usual drugs given to alleviate anxiety, stress and insomnia. Most doctors had considerable reservations about them, so when the benzodiazepines were introduced in the 1970s it was thought that a safe alternative had been found. Accordingly, there was a complete switch to the prescription of benzodiazepine drugs.

At the present time in 1993, about 3 per cent of the British population will have been taking a benzodiazepine drug regularly over the preceding year. Some 60 per cent of these prescriptions will be for sleeping tablets.

At the moment there are nine benzodiazepines which are prescribable on the NHS. In addition, others are available on production of a private prescription from a medical practitioner.

Although the drugs are marketed as being either hypnotics (sleeping tablets) or anxiolytics (tranquillizers), the differentiation is irrelevant. The truth is that all of the benzodiazepines have both hypnotic and anxiolytic actions.

It has to be said that these drugs are extremely effective at relieving anxiety and improving sleep when given over a short period of time. If they are taken for too long, however (which could be as little as a fortnight), then a physical and psychological dependence is liable to develop.

The main problems with taking them long term are that they cause drowsiness and reduce one's reaction time. They can alter mood, affect one's perception abilities, and sometimes they end up worsening the conditions they were prescribed for in the first place.

It is desirable to stop them if possible. Because there are problems with withdrawal, however, this should be done slowly under medical supervision. In addition, support from friends, people who have experienced a similar problem, and advice from groups such as MIND and TRANX are well worth seeking.

UNDER NO CIRCUMSTANCES SHOULD ONE SUDDENLY STOP TAKING TRANQUILLISERS OR SLEEPING TABLETS, WITHOUT FIRST CONSULTING YOUR DOCTOR. THE CONSEQUENCES OF DOING SO COULD BE SERIOUS AND DANGEROUS.

Homoeopathic remedies can be helpful. I feel that the constitutional remedy is the best first step, although if it cannot easily be traced, then one can consider remedies appropriate for the condition it was prescribed for (See relevant chapters), or one of the following.

Arsenicum album – for fussy, restless types, prone to regularly recurring problems.

Calcarea carbonica – for slow, congested types who are worse for mental or physical exertion.

Capsicum – for peevish types who are prone to homesickness. They may be 'peppery.' They tend to crave stimulants and can easily become dependent on medication.

Ignatia – for hysterical types who may suffer illness after grief or strong emotions.

Nux vomica – for fiery, irritable types who are prone to use all sorts of stimulants.

Sepia – for indifferent, melancholic types who can be lifted out of themselves if encouraged to do some favourite activity.

Twitches and Tics

Nervous mannerisms, facial tics, grunts and groans are all difficult to master. A tic may occur several times a minute, every minute of every waking hour. They can completely dominate one's life. Attempts to stop them can work for short periods, but there is always a great amount of tension generated.

Distraction and channelling of one's energies into some intricate process might help.

Aconite – if a twitch has developed after an acute shock, fright or trauma.

Argentum nitricum – for twitches in anxious types who tend to get diarrhoea in anticipation of an event. Their twitch may also become more obvious when they are stressed.

Arsenicum album – for twitches in tidy, fussy, restless types.

Cuprum metallicum – for nervous spasms and twitches. May have a coppery taste in the mouth.

Gelsemium – for twitches and tremors when frightened or acutely stressed. They generally 'shake like a leaf' when frightened.

Phosphorus – for twitches in artistic, creative types.

Thuja occidentalis – for twitches in hurried, sensitive types who tend to develop fixed ideas. They may have a tendency to develop warts.

Zincum metallicum – for twitches and tremors in slow, melancholic types who tend to repeat things said to them.

CHAPTER 18

Shock, Trauma and Abuse

Many ailments and illnesses have their origin at a time of great upset, be that physical, emotional, or a mixture of the two. Indeed, some would suggest that a traumatic birth alone can cause such a shock to the whole being that they enter the world in a congenitally wounded emotional state. Their whole subsequent development, as they learn about themselves and the world about them, may be faulty because of the shaky foundation they have been given to build upon.

Other 'primal' injuries can cause blocks, or aberrations in the vibration of the etheric body, thereby resulting in emotional troubles or physical ailments. The way we are today is a result of all that has happened to us up to that point in time.

Orthodox opinion would accept that scars and past illnesses may have an effect upon the functioning of the human body. Physical traumas can affect the structural integrity of the body to reduce function, and psychological shocks can affect our mental reasoning. No-one would argue with that.

Homoeopathy goes further than that and suggests that all things affect the individual, but that compensating mechanisms allow for functioning to continue. While old infections may be cured, they often leave a legacy, a sort of shadow of the original problem. Similarly, emotional blows can be 'overcome' yet continue to exert an effect upon the vibration of the individual. These problems can be likened to the building up of layers of a pearl or an onion, each layer representing a trauma, event or illness which contributes to the whole of the individual.

Understand, however, that although I have described them as individual layers, they are actually vibrational patterns, rather than shells. As such, they continue to exert an effect since they are in a constant state of 'oneness' with the whole self. Not only that, but a new emotional assault, trauma or event can suddenly produce an alteration in the vibrational pattern to cause a release of one of the vibrational layers, hence producing a flare-up of a past problem. That in turn may alter the vibrational nature of other layers to cause other symptoms to occur.

The reality is that the individual is a complicated vibrational interference pattern, a composite of all his past physical and emotional experiences.

Homoeopathic remedies can be extremely useful in helping the individual deal with acute emotional shock, the associated shock after physical trauma, and with the deep-rooted long-term effects of past shock, trauma and abuse.

Acute Shock

Under this heading I include the ill effects of bad news, personal tragedy or severe fright.

Aconite – for restlessness and agitation and panic with acute shock. They may develop a fever as a result. The old-fashioned attack of 'brain fever' following an emotional blow.

Ignatia – for an acute hysterical reaction after a shock. There may be acute asthma, hysterical overbreathing or even a type of 'fit.'

Lycopodium – for irritability and extreme sensitivity after a shock. There is a great fear that they might 'snap' and have a breakdown.

Natrum muriaticum – for migraine with a hammering headache and zig-zag vision after a shock. May slip into tearful depression, although will be worse for consolation. Will want to be on their own to let the emotions out.

Opium – for shock which may have caused loss of consciousness. They cannot grasp things after the event.

Phosphoric acidum – for shock in mild, amiable types. They become completely indifferent to everything. Literally, too-shocked to react. May develop some illness as a result.

Phosphorus – for shock in artistic, creative types who are very sensitive to atmospheres.

Pulsatilla – for shock in timid, shy types who are generally better for being outdoors. When shocked they may need to get to the air.

ACUTE SHOCK WITH PHYSICAL TRAUMA

Under this heading I think of the ill effects upon the emotions caused by physical injury.

Aconite – for restlessness, agitation and panic after a trauma. May become quite fevered.

Arnica – called 'the healer.' A superb remedy for the ill effects of all accidents. Can remove the shock perhaps years after the incident occurred.

Carbo vegetabilis – a great remedy when there is severe trauma and the individual is extremely weak. Medical aid is imperative, but a dose of this remedy may be life-saving. It is a remedy for the glove-compartment of the car or the medicine cabinet.

Hypericum – for the shock which occurs when nerves are crushed or concussed. Ideal for the fingers trapped in doors, eye injuries or bad penetrating injuries.

Opium – for shock which may have caused loss of consciousness. They cannot grasp things after the event.

Past Shock and Abuse

One of the most tragic and psychologically damaging things which can happen to a person is to be sexually abused. The effects last for the whole of life and all sorts of emotions tend to flare up. It is the classical case of mixed emotional problems.

Because of the enormity of the trauma, the violation of the individual's body, the betrayal of trust, the fear, threats and all that goes with such a heinous crime, it is perhaps a mercy that the human mind is able to suppress much of the memory.

Or so one might think!

The truth is that although the mind can suppress or repress the memory of the actual event (perhaps!) the effects continue to gnaw away at the victim. Fear usually lies at the very core of the problem, coupled with guilt, lack of self-esteem, depressive episodes and possible self-destructive thoughts. Imagine the sheer horror of living with these emotions when there is no obvious memory of why this should be the case.

Sexual abuse of another human being destroys their life!

IF THERE IS ANY SUSPICION THAT A SEXUAL ABUSE HAS TAKEN PLACE THEN MEDICAL HELP SHOULD BE SOUGHT.

Homoeopathic remedies may be helpful. The use of **Arnica** or **Aconite** might be valuable in alleviating the original shock. The other emotions are worth looking at separately and treating one at a time. For example, if guilt is the predominant feeling then the remedy corresponding best to that guilt pattern would be the first remedy. Then the feeling of fear – specific, anticipatory, or free-floating, may need to be handled. Finally, the depression could be focused upon.

This particular problem is sadly extremely common in most cultures. It is difficult to treat, so the help of a professional is vital.

Part Three

Notes on Taking
The Remedies
Materia Medica
Therapeutic Index

Taking the Remedies

It is important to remember the following points when taking Homoeopathic remedies in tablet form.

*The tablets should not be handled, but should be flicked into the mouth from the lid of the container, or placed there with a spoon. This is because the effectiveness of the tablet is only on the surface, not mixed all the way through as is a conventional tablet.

*Two tablets should be taken at a time – but they must be sucked not swallowed.

*The tablets should not be taken within half an hour of tea, food, coffee, smoking or having brushed the teeth.

*The remedies will last for a long time, providing they are kept away from potent smelling substances. They are best kept in a drawer, away from perfumes, spices, pot-pouri or moth-balls.

Two potencies are recommended – 30C and 200C. Both potencies may be available from chemists who stock homoeopathic remedies, health food shops, or directly from homoeopathic suppliers (See useful addresses at the back of the book). The 30C should suffice for all the problems covered, although the 200C being a higher potency is likely to have a more intense effect in the realm of the emotions.

If the constitutional remedy is obvious from a study of the Materia Medica then this can be taken in 30C potency, two tablets three times a day at the start of any acute disturbance.

It should only be taken for three days. If improvement starts within that time then the remedy should be stopped then and there. There is no point whatsoever in '*taking extra just to make sure.*' It should not be repeated unless the symptoms reappear.

If a problem seems to be related to the menstrual cycle (See the Chapter on Premenstrual Syndrome) then I find it is best to take the remedies for the three days after the period has stopped.

The constitutional remedy can also be taken for three days at a time every three months as a booster.

If a high potency remedy is taken continuously for too long (more than three days) then there is a strong likelihood of producing an aggravation of symptoms.

Low potency remedies, eg 6C, are less good than the high potencies when dealing with emotional problems, but they do have an advantage in that they can be taken more frequently. However, it should again be appreciated that they should be stopped once symptomatic improvement occurs. They should not be repeated unless the symptoms start to come back. Their best place in treatment seems to be when dealing with the outer layers of mixed emotions (See Chapter on Mixed Emotions).

Materia medica

This covers the remedy profiles of all the remedies included in this book.

As you will see, I have considered each remedy under the headings of mentals, modalities, likes and dislikes, physical features, together with their disease and emotional tendencies, as discussed in Chapter 3. Characteristic features of the remedies will be emphasised in capital letters, eg the THIRST of Aconite.

The major 'Constitutional' remedies will be marked with an asterisk.

Although there are many, many more remedies which are of value in emotional problems, I have restricted the number to avoid making the book too complicated, yet tried to ensure that the most useful ones (in my experience) are included.

MATERIA MEDICA

The following remedies are used throughout this book.

Remedy	*Abbreviation*
Aconite	Acon
Alumina	Alum
Ammonium bromatum	Ammon br
Ammonium carbonicum	Ammon carb
Anacardium orientale	Anac
Apis mellifica	Apis
Argentum nitricum	Arg nit
Arnica	Arn
Arsenicum album	Ars alb
Arum triphyllum	Arum tri
Aurum metallicum	Aur

Baryta carbonica	Bar carb
Belladonna	Bell
Bryonia	Bry
Cactus grandiflorus	Cact
Calcarea carbonica	Calc carb
Calcarea phosphorica	Calc phos
Capsicum	Cap
Carbo vegetabilis	Carb veg
Causticum	Caust
Chamomilla	Cham
China officinalis	Chin
Cimicifuga	Cimic
Cina	Cina
Cocculus	Cocc
Coffea	Coff
Colocynth	Coloc
Cuprum metallicum	Cup met
Equisetum	Equis
Gelsemium	Gels
Graphites	Graph
Hepar sulph	Hep sulph
Hyoscyamus	Hyos
Hypericum	Hyper
Ignatia	Ign
Iodum	Iod
Kali phos	Kali phos
Lachesis	Lach
Lilium tigrinum	Lil tig
Lycopodium	Lyc
Mercurius solubilis	Merc
Natrum carbonicum	Nat carb
Natrum muriaticum	Nat mur
Nitricum acidum	Nit ac
Nux vomica	Nux vom
Opium	Op
Phosphoricum acidum	Phos ac
Phosphorus	Phos
Picric acidum	Pic ac
Platina	Plat
Pulsatilla	Puls

Rhododendron	Rhod
Rhus toxicodendron	Rhus tox
Sabadilla	Sabad
Sepia	Sep
Silicea	Sil
Spigelia	Spig
Staphisagria	Staph
Stramonium	Stram
Sulphur	Sulph
Tarentula hispania	Tarent
Thuja occidentalis	Thuj
Valerian	Valer
Veratrum album	Verat
Zincum metallicum	Zinc

ACONITE
(Monkshood)

A good remedy for THE START OF ILLNESSES. Not very good for chronic illness.
Always RESTLESS.
THIRST becomes marked.
TINGLING, NUMBNESS of local parts and BURNING internal pains.

Mentals
Great fear and anxiety with any illness.
Forebodings of doom.
Fear of death, darkness and ghosts.
Anxiety about the future.
Becomes restless.
Good imagination.
May feel clairvoyant.

Modalities
Better for open air.
Worse in warm rooms.
Worse in evenings and night.
Worse on getting out of bed.

Worse for dry, cold winds and draughts.
Worse for music.

Likes and dislikes

Thirst for cold water.

Physical features

Robust, good coloured types.

Disease tendencies

Eye inflammations.
Feverish illnesses brought on by shock, fright, draughts, and too much sun.

Emotional tendencies

Panic.
Agoraphobia.
Phobias of darkness, death and ghosts.
Fixed ideas and obsessions.
Anger with shock.
Alcohol dependence.
Nervous twitches and tics.
Acute shock producing a feverish illness, the old-fashioned 'brain fever.'
Acute shock with traumas.
Insomnia and night-mares.

ALUMINA

(Aluminium oxide)

Alumina is a remedy against the toxic effects of aluminium.
There is general DRYNESS of mucus membranes.
There is WEAKNESS or even PARALYSIS of parts.
There is general SLUGGISHNESS of all functions.

Mentals

Variable mood, but with slight tendency towards melancholia.
Fear that will lose the power of reason.
Memory problems and poor concentration.
Always hurried, although time seems to drag.

Modalities
Worse in the mornings.
Worse for warm rooms.
Worse for eating potatoes.
Better for open air.
Better for damp weather.
Better one day, worse on the next.

Likes and dislikes
Unusual tastes for indigestible things.
Likes tea and coffee.
Likes fruit and vegetables.
Dislikes meat.
Dislikes potatoes.

Physical features
Pale, dry and possibly cracked skin.
Thin builds.

Disease tendencies
Dry eyes.
Dryness of the membranes of the respiratory system, with cough, chronic catarrh and hoarseness.
Headaches over top of skull.
Constipation with hard knotty motions.
Dry, cracked, itching skin problems.
Itching of back passage.
Numbness, weakness and paralysis of limbs.
Paralytic states.

Emotional tendencies
Chronic Fatigue Syndrome.
Anorexia.
Loss of appetite.

AMMONIUM BROMATUM
(Ammonium Bromide)

Does not have many mental symptoms.
DRY, SPASMODIC COUGHS.

TICKLING THROAT.

Emotional tendencies

Nail-biting. There is a feeling of itching at the fingertips and under the nails. The only relief is from biting the nails.

AMMONIUM CARBONICUM

(Ammonium carbonate)

Mainly a female remedy.

Well-nourished women who lead sedentary lives.

SLOWNESS in all things.

AVERSION TO WATER – DISLIKE OF WASHING AND BATHING.

Mentals

Forgetfulness.

Gloomy during stormy weather.

Sad and weepy.

Uncleanliness.

Modalities

Worse in evenings.

Worse for washing, bathing.

Better for dry weather.

Likes and dislikes

Increased appetite for most things.

Physical features

Tendency to avoid washing.

Cracked corners of mouth.

Disease tendencies

Heavy periods.

Tonsillitis and glandular problems.

Emotional tendencies

Chronic Fatigue Syndrome.

Post Viral Debility.

Bulimia.
Increased appetite.

ANACARDIUM ORIENTALE
(Marking Nut)

Mentals
Useful for MEMORY LOSS.
Irritable and angry with unusual and unexpected SWEARING.
May have strong moral sense, so feel GUILTY.
Have a tendency to develop strange fixations. For example, may feel as if he is two people, or that he is possessed.
Easily offended.

Modalities
Better for lying on painful part.
Better for rubbing.
Better for eating.
Worse for heat.
Worse for washing or bathing with hot water.

Likes and dislikes
Likes milk and dairy products.

Physical features
Pale face.
Blue rings around the eyes.

Disease tendencies
Sensations of a PLUG in the back passage, in the ear, in the nose.
May get dyspepsia of the stomach, better for eating.
May get intense ITCHING of the skin which makes the irritability worse.
DIMINUTION OF ALL SENSES.

Emotional tendencies
Peculiar fixations and obsessive-compulsive behaviour, particularly in the elderly.

Memory problems.
Over-sensitivity, irritability and anger.
Unexpected swearing.
Hate.
Guilt.
Nervous exhaustion.

APIS MELLIFICA
(The Honey-Bee)

Useful when there is sudden SWELLING or PUFFINESS of tissues which comes on suddenly.
BURNING and STINGING and THROBBING pains.
Very TENDER and SENSITIVE to touch.
ABSENT THIRST.

Mentals
Apathy and indifference.
Fear of death
Memory problems.
Jealousy.
Tearfulness.
Whining.
Hard to please.
Clumsiness.

Modalities
Worse for heat in any form.
Worse for touch and pressure.
Worse for sleep.
Better for uncovering and for cold water.

Likes and dislikes
Craving for milk.

Disease tendencies
Headaches, which stab and sting and are worse for movement.
Eye problems which sting and burn.
Spasmodic cough.

Itching skin. May have wheals like nettle rash.
Acute flare-ups of arthritis which sting and burn.
Insect stings.
Urinary incontinence with stinging as the urine is passed.

Emotional tendencies
Apathy.
Indifference.
Fear of death.
Jealousy.

ARGENTUM NITRICUM *****
(Silver nitrate)

ANXIETY and APPREHENSION.
SPLINTER-LIKE SENSATIONS.

Mentals
Anticipatory fear. Will worry for days before an engagement, appointment or event.
The anxiety causes DIARRHOEA.
Fear of death.
Fear of heights with Lemming impulse, as if would like to jump off.
Fear of insects and spiders.
Claustrophobia.
Sexual fears.
Fixed ideas and strange compulsions. May feel compelled to do things for reasons which may be logical to them, but which they know would seem strange to anyone else.
Never feels that there is enough time. Always in a hurry.

Modalities
Worse for heat.
Worse at night.
Worse for sweet things.
Worse for getting into any emotional state.
Better for belching.
Better for cold air.

Better for pressure.
Worse for concentration.

Likes and dislikes

Craves sweets and chocolate.
Likes salt.
Likes cheese.

Physical features

Thin builds. May suit extroverted types who achieve because they fear failure so much. May wonder why they put themselves in certain situations as they anticipate the event or whatever with fear, trepidation and diarrhoea.

Disease tendencies

Eyestrain.
Flatulence.
Diarrhoea.
Splinter-like sore throats and splinter-like pains.
Anxiety states.
HEADACHES with TREMBLING, worse for concentration.
TREMBLING and weakness of lower limbs.

Emotional tendencies

Anticipatory fear and fear of performing.
Claustrophobia.
Fear of insects and spiders.
Fear of death.
Fear of heights.
Sexual fears in males.
Impulsive and tendency to follow strange impulses.
Fixed ideas.
Bulimia.
Increased appetite and craving for chocolate.
Bed-wetting.
Nail-biting.
Twitches and tics.

Arnica
(Leopard's Bane)

AFTER TRAUMA.
SORE, BRUISED FEELINGS.
SHOCK AFTER INJURY OR ACCIDENT.
A good first aid remedy, called 'Arnica the healer.'

Mentals
Indifferent.
Irritable.
Forgetful and absent-minded.
Fear of death.
GREAT FEAR OF BEING TOUCHED when in pain.
Always says he feels well, even if very ill.

Modalities
Worse for touch.
Worse for motion.
Worse for damp.
Worse for alcohol.
BETTER FOR LYING DOWN.

Likes and dislikes
Likes pickles.
Likes vinegar.
Dislike of meat.
Dislike of milk.

Physical features
Maybe slightly melancholic. Generally stoical types who minimise problems and dislike bothering their doctors.

Disease tendencies
All traumas.
Will remove the shock created by an accident or injury, even if this happened years in the past. Chronic problems arising from that shock may clear up after treatment with Arnica.

Emotional tendencies

Agoraphobia.

Insomnia – the bed always feels too hard.

Acute trauma and shock.

ARSENICUM ALBUM *****

(Arsenic)

There is very marked FASTIDIOUSNESS.

There is PERIODICITY of symptoms (eg, symptoms tend to recur at regular intervals).

There are BURNING PAINS.

RESTLESSNESS is marked.

There is CHILLINESS.

Right-sided problems.

Mentals

There is anxiety and anguish.

There may be hypochondriasis.

With illness there may be hopelessness, as if the feeling is that nothing can help.

The reaction is out of proportion to the condition and irritability may be the result.

May need to take to bed for the slightest of problems.

There is restlessness and agitation.

Agoraphobia.

Fear of burglars, death and ghosts.

Soon exhausted.

NEAT in all things. Almost OBSESSIONAL. Appearance, clothes, house and garden – they all have to be tended and groomed.

Thirsty.

Modalities

Worse for wet weather.

WORSE AROUND MIDNIGHT UNTIL 2AM

Worse for cold, cold drinks or food.

Better for heat.

Better for warm drinks.

Likes and dislikes

Likes fat.

Likes small drinks.

Physical features

Anxious, pale and thin. Intelligent, quick-witted and perfectionist types.

Disease tendencies

Skin problems, psoriasis, dandruff, heart failure, watery head colds which cause sore red noses.

Emotional tendencies

Restless fear.

Agoraphobia.

Fear of burglars, death, darkness and ghosts.

Fixed ideas and obsessions.

Hypochondriasis.

Agitated depression.

Grief reaction.

Irritability.

Jealousy.

Guilt.

Insomnia.

Alcohol dependence.

Thumb-sucking.

Tobacco addiction.

Twitches and tics.

ARUM TRIPHYLLUM

(Jack-in-the-Pulpit)

ACRID, EXCORIATING DISCHARGES.

There are not many mental symptoms with this remedy.

There is a tendency to do things until they bleed.

Emotional tendencies

Nail-biting.

Nose-picking, as if 'boring' into the nose. Often may have small nose-bleeds as a result.

AURUM METALLICUM
(Gold)

AILMENTS CAUSED BY GRIEF.
There is CHILLINESS.
BORING PAINS.

Mentals
LACK OF CONFIDENCE.
AGITATED DEPRESSION, possibly even suicidal.
Extreme sensitivity.
There may be hypochondriasis.
Fixed ideas and obsessions about suicide and death.
Hate contradiction.
Irritability and anger.
CRITICAL of everyone and everything.
Prefers own company and dislikes having to talk.
Noises cause anxiety.
Fear of men.
Often troubled with nightmares.
Guilt.
Hate.

Modalities
Worse at night.
Worse for concentration.
Worse on waking.
Better for cold.
May get problems in Winter – 'Seasonal Affective Disorder,' known as SAD.

Likes and dislikes
Craves alcohol.

Physical features
May have a staring, melancholic appearance.

Disease tendencies
Catarrhal problems.
Nose and ear problems.

Boring and tearing joint and bone pains.
Skin ulcers.

Emotional tendencies

Fixed ideas and obsessions, often about suicide.
Hypochondriasis.
Agitated depression.
Grief reactions.
Over-sensitivity.
Irritability.
Guilt.
Hate.
Problems from disappointed love or relationship problems.
Anorexia.
Loss of appetite and loathing of body image.
Menopausal problems and post-menopausal depression.

BARYTA CARBONICA *****

(Barium carbonate)

There is often ENLARGEMENT of GLANDS, cysts, lipomas (fatty lumps), nodules and the PROSTATE GLAND in men.
There is CHILLINESS.

Mentals

There is memory loss and difficulty thinking.
Tendency to dwell on problems and past grievances.
Fear of things about to happen.
Fear of strangers.
Confusion.

Modalities

WORSE FOR THINKING ABOUT PROBLEMS.
Worse for washing.
Worse lying on affected side.
Better in open air.

Likes and dislikes

Cold food.

Physical features

Tendency to be overweight.
Dry wrinkled skin.

Disease tendencies

Headaches which feel as if the brain is loose.
Recurrent sore throats with enlarged glands.
Lipomas and cysts.
Dry coughs.
Palpitations when lying on left.
Constipation with hard knobbly motions.
Haemorrhoids which come out when urine is passed.
Urinary frequency.
Prostate problems.

Emotional tendencies

Fear of strangers.
Memory problems.
Confusional states, particularly in the elderly.

BELLADONNA

(Deadly Nightshade)

There is HOTNESS, REDNESS, THROBBING and BURNING.
It is an acute remedy.
There is no thirst.
The ailment comes on rapidly.
Right-sided problems.

> ALL OF THESE FEATURES CAN BE THE RESULT OF A SEVERE BACTERIAL INFECTION AND NEED TO BE CHECKED OUT BY A PROFESSIONAL. THIS IS IMPORTANT BECAUSE SO MANY DANGEROUS INFECTIONS CAN START THIS WAY.

Mentals

May seem delirious.
May be angry or furious.
All the senses seem to be acute.

Guilt.
Agitated depression.

Modalities
Worse for touch.
Worse for being jarred.
Worse for noise.
Worse for draughts.
Better sitting up.
Better for warm room.

Likes and dislikes
Dislike of meat.
Dislike of milk.
Worse for having a haircut.
Worse for getting head cold.

Physical features
Strong types.
Vivacious when well, but knocked for six when ill and seem to go delirious.

Disease tendencies
All sudden infections, as mentioned above. It can be used usefully as an adjunct to orthodox treatment.
Throbbing headaches.

Emotional tendencies
Agitated depression.
Irritability with quick outbursts of 'hot' temper. May go red in the face.
Guilt.
Insomnia from restless legs.
Vaginismus.

BRYONIA
(Wild Hop)

DRYNESS runs through this remedy. There are dry mucus membranes, dry mouth, dry eyes, dry coughs and hard dry motions.

Right-sided complaints.
STITCHING AND TEARING PAINS.
AILMENTS BROUGHT ON BY ANGER.
Excessive thirst.

Mentals
There is IRRITABILITY and anger.
Desires to be left alone when ill.
Poor memory.
Fear of death.
Restless fear.

Modalities
WORSE FOR MOVEMENT of any kind.
WORSE FOR COLD WINDS.
Better for cold.
Better for being perfectly still.
All ailments better for pressure, except abdominal problems which are made worse.
Better for lying on painful side.
Ailments may start with first of the warm weather.

Physical features
Dark skin and dark haired (or previously so).
Good build, but not obese.

Disease tendencies
Headaches of a splitting or bursting nature. Better for pressure.
Arthritis and rheumatic pains which are better for being still.
Constipation.
Dry coughs and pleurisy.

Emotional tendencies
Restless fear.
Fear of death.
Irritability.

Cactus Grandiflorus
(Night-blooming Cereus)

Produces CONSTRICTING and VICE-LIKE pains.
Ailments tend to be PERIODIC, or come at regular intervals.

Mentals
Melancholic.
Anxiety.
Pains are so bad that feels like screaming.
Sexual fears.

Modalities
Worse lying on left side.
Better in open air.
Better for pressure.

Disease tendencies
Headaches which are vice-like.
Angina pains which are vice-like.
Palpitations when walking.

Emotional problems
Vaginismus.

Calcarea Carbonica *****
(Calcium carbonate)

There is CHILLINESS.
There is SLOWNESS.
There is CONGESTION of all types – of the heart, lungs, bowels.
There is SOFTNESS.

Mentals
Restless fear.
ALL SORTS OF FEARS – of the dark, impending doom, insanity and death.
Fear of strokes is common.
Anxiety worse in the evenings, producing palpitations.

Lethargic depression.
Forgetfulness and confusion.
Forget what they have read soon after putting the book or magazine aside.
There is general slowness of thought.
There is a tendency to dwell on problems, often to the exasperation of friends and relatives.
Talking about their problems makes them weep.
Dislike criticism or hard talking, which makes them anxious.
Jealousy.
Hate.

Modalities

WORSE FOR EXERTION – both physical and mental.
Worse for the cold in every form.
Worse for the damp.
Worse for standing.
Worse during the full moon.
Better for dryness and warm weather.
Better for lying on painful side.
Better for rubbing.
Better for lying on back.

Likes and dislikes

Dislikes meat.
Dislikes boiled food.
Dislikes fat.
Dislikes milk.
Likes indigestible things.
Likes eggs.
Likes salt.
Likes sweets.

Physical features

There is a flabby, doughy, soft appearance.
The handshake is floppy and the knuckles of the hands may appear as dimples, because of the soft, doughy appearance.
The feet tend to be cold and clammy.
There is a tendency to sweat on the head and chest.

Disease tendencies
Chronic catarrh (Congestion).
Nasal polyps (Congestion).
Dry irritating cough (Congestion).
Constipation (Congestion).
Warts.
Obesity.
Backache.

Emotional tendencies
Restless fear.
Fear of dark, death, insanity.
Hypochondriasis.
Lethargic or retarded depression.
Jealousy.
Hate.
Chronic Fatigue Syndrome.
Bulimia.
Premenstrual Syndrome (PMS).

CALCAREA PHOSPHORICA
(Calcium Phosphate)

Delayed tooth development in childhood.
Poor bone healing.
NUMBNESS and CRAWLING PAINS.

Mentals
Poor memory.
Peevish.
AILMENTS AND ILLNESS STARTING AFTER DISAPPOINTED LOVE.

Modalities
Worse in damp.
Worse in cold and snow.
Better in the dry. Better for warmth.

Likes and dislikes
Craves salt and salty foods.

Physical features
Small build, although may be stout.
Usually dark.

Disease tendencies
Bone disorders.
Poor healing.

Emotional tendencies
Ailments coming on after disappointed love, or unrequited love.

CAPSICUM
(Cayenne pepper)

OBESITY
Wounds tend to supperate.
Burning pains.

Mentals
Peevish.
Irritability with 'peppery' temper.
Uncleanliness.
HOMESICKNESS.

Modalities
Worse for washing.
Worse for being uncovered.
Better for heat.
Better while eating.

Likes and dislikes
Craves all sorts of stimulants.
Thirsty.

Physical features
Obese, lethargic, unclean.
Tendency to have spots.

Emotional tendencies
Irritability and anger.
Homesickness.
Stimulants overuse.

CARBO VEGETABILIS
(Vegetable charcoal)

Chronic complaints.
An excellent remedy when there is profound weakness or physical shock.

Mentals
Memory loss.
Fear of strangers.
Fear of enclosed spaces.

Modalities
Worse in the evenings.
Worse for the cold.
Better for fanning.

Likes and dislikes
Dislike of fats.
Dislike of meat.
Dislike of milk.

Physical features
Overweight, lethargic and with tendency to bloat. May feel hot and in need of fanning. Mottling of the cheeks with a red nose.

Disease tendencies
Extreme exhaustion with shock or after prolonged illness.
Nose-bleeds.
Bloated abdomen and digestive problems.
Hoarseness.

Emotional tendencies
Claustrophobia.
Fear of strangers.
Acute shock.

Causticum *****
(Potassium hydrate)

BURNING, BURSTING and TEARING PAINS.
PROGRESSIVE WEAKNESS leading to PARALYSIS.
Contractures.
Conditions caused by grief.

Mentals
Fear of animals, darkness, death, ghosts, strangers, performing.
Despair of recovery.
Fear of the dark.
Fear of doom.
Irritability.
Bereavement may cause illness.
Sympathetic to others.
Poor memory.
Concentration makes symptoms worse.

Modalities
WORSE FOR COLD WINDS
Worse for motion.
Better in damp, warm weather.

Likes and dislikes
Upset by smell of food.
Worse for sweet foods.
Worse for coffee.

Physical features
Broken-down appearance – sickly looking, dark eyed types who are 'rheumatic.'
Dark hair.

Disease tendencies
Paralytic problems, especially when single nerves are affected, eg Bell's palsy (Facial palsy).
Contractures of muscles and tendons.
Painful neck, brought on by the cold.
Tearing pains of muscles, joints and bones.

Stress incontinence, when coughing, sneezing, laughing and exertion cause urine to be passed involuntarily.
Haemorrhoids.
Warts, especially on the face and fingers.

Emotional tendencies
Bottled-up fear.
Fears of animals, darkness, death, ghosts, strangers, performing.
Grief reaction.
Guilt.
Ailments from disappointed love or unrequited love.
Anorexia.
Premenstrual Syndrome (PMS).

CHAMOMILLA
(Chamomile)

Mentals
Irritability and anger.
Whining is common.
Impatience.
Spiteful and snappy.
Angry when in pain.

Modalities
Worse for heat.
Worse for anger.
Better for being carried (children).
Better for warm, wet weather.

Likes and dislikes
Nothing seems to satisfy them.
Nauseated after coffee.

Physical features
One cheek may be red and hot.
Very restless.
A child is always wanting to be picked up and cannot be placated.

Disease tendencies
Earache, toothache, all severe infective pain conditions.

Emotional tendencies
Anger and irritability.
Over-sensitivity to everything.

CHINA OFFICINALIS
(Cinchona bark)

A remedy for DEBILITY – from diarrhoea, blood loss, excess perspiration and excessive use of laxatives (ie from loss of body fluids).
PERIODICITY – complaints often come every other day.
There is CHILLINESS.

Mentals
Apathy.
Indifference.
Despair.
Fears of animals and 'creepie-crawlies.'
Can be deliberately hurtful to others when the mood takes them.
Thoughts whirl around the mind, causing insomnia.
Sudden, unexpected bursts of tears.

Modalities
WORSE FOR SLIGHTEST TOUCH.
Worse every other day.
Worse for losing fluids from the body.
Better for doubling up.
BETTER FOR FIRM PRESSURE.
Better for the open air.
Better for warmth.

Likes and dislikes
Dislikes milk.
Dislikes fruit.

Physical features

Hollow eyed, blue rings around them and a yellow appearance to the sclera (BUT NOT JAUNDICE – it is not something which develops, but an appearance which has always been present).
Sweats around the nose.

Disease tendencies

BURSTING HEADACHES followed by TENDER SCALP, RELIEVED BY PRESSURE.
Abdominal distension not relieved by passing wind.
TINNITUS (ringing in ears) – sensitive to touch.
DEAFNESS associated with the tinnitus.

Emotional tendencies

Fears of animals and 'creepie-crawlies'.
Lethargic or retarded depression.
Irritability.
Chronic Fatigue Syndrome.
Post Viral Debility or exhaustion.
Insomnia.
Bulimia after an illness when there has been loss of vital fluids.

CIMICIFUGA

(Black Snake-root)

Mainly a female remedy.
MUSCULAR AND CRAMP PAINS.
AGITATION AND PAIN.

Mentals

Cloud of depression seems to descend.
Feelings of impending doom.
Hysterical outbursts.
Self-destructive behaviour.

Modalities

Worse during a menstrual period.
Worse in the morning.
Worse for the cold.

Better for warmth.
Better after food.

Likes and dislikes
Nil in particular.

Physical features
Nil in particular.

Disease tendencies
Gynaecological pains with agitation.
Muscular pains and 'rheumatism.'
Neuralgia.

Emotional tendencies
Hysterical depression.
Self-destructive outbursts.
Hysterical outbursts.
Dreams of impending evil.
Depression after unsuccessful romances.

CINA
(Worm-seed)

Usually a children's remedy.
SKIN SENSITIVITY.

Mentals
Irritability.
Cross and doesn't want to be touched, or carried.
Cannot be satisfied.

Emotional tendencies
Nose-picking. The nose itches and the child can only seem to relieve it by picking it.
Teeth-grinding.

Cocculus
(Indian cockle)

DEBILITY FROM LACK OF SLEEP.
Good remedy for travel-sickness and VERTIGO
There is a sense of HOLLOWNESS of affected parts.
There is a sense of the affected parts having GONE TO SLEEP.

Mentals
CAPRICIOUS.
Gets very sad.
Bursts into song.
Slow on the uptake sometimes.
Fast speech.
Concerned for others.
SENSITIVE TO INSULTS OR CONTRADICTION.
Difficulty thinking and concentrating if has missed sleep.
Unable to find the right word.
Guilt.

Modalities
WORSE FOR EATING.
NAUSEA AT THE SMELL OF FOOD, especially when has vertigo.
WORSE FOR LACK OF SLEEP.
WORSE FOR MOTION.
Worse after emotional upset.

Likes and dislikes
Likes cold beer.
When nauseated, dislikes all food.

Physical features
Often some lameness, paralysis or weakness.
May be light haired.

Disease tendencies
Painful contractures of the limbs, especially when affecting one side of the body.
Numbness of parts, as if they've gone to sleep.

Facial paralysis.
Constant drowsiness with spasmodic yawning.

Emotional tendencies
Over-anxious about others.
Guilt.

COFFEA
(Coffee)

There is HYPERSENSITIVITY to pain.
All pains seem intolerable.
There is abnormal activity of the brain. Mind-buzz.
Neuralgias.

Mentals
There is irritability.
The senses seem acute.
The mind buzzes with ideas.
Anxiety also comes swiftly and produces restlessness and anguish.
Insomnia because of the mind-buzz.
Guilt.

Modalities
WORSE FOR EXCESS EMOTIONS OF ALL SORTS (eg excitement, anger joy).
Worse for strong smells.
Worse for open air.
Better for warmth.
Better for lying down.
Better for holding cold water in mouth.

Physical features
Tall, lean types with a tendency to stoop.
Dark complexion.

Disease tendencies
HEADACHES LIKE A NAIL BEING DRIVEN INTO SKULL.
Palpitations when excited, overjoyed or angry.
Hypersensitive skin.

Emotional tendencies
Guilt.
Insomnia or migraine after unsuccessful love.

COLOCYNTH
(Bitter cucumber)

Ailments which follow ANGER or INDIGNATION.
Often causes intense NEURALGIAS.
CRAMPING, CUTTING, CONSTRICTING and SPASM pains.
Agonising, DOUBLING-UP abdominal pains.
Symptoms often start on the LEFT SIDE.

Mentals
Restlessness.
Irritability.
Angry when questioned.
Indignation.
Quick to take offence.

Modalities
WORSE FOR ANGER.
Worse for indignation.
BETTER FOR DOUBLING-UP.
Better for hard pressure.

Likes and dislikes
Dislikes cheese.

Physical features
Tendency to be overweight.
Offensive smelling perspiration.
Contracted muscles.

Disease tendencies
Neuralgias – mainly LEFT-SIDED.
Sciatica – left sided.
Cramps relieved by lying on the affected side with the legs drawn up.

Emotional tendencies
Irritability.
Indignation.
Ailments developing with suppressed anger or after anger.

CUPRUM METALLICUM
(Copper)

CRAMPING, CONSTRICTING and SPASM pains.
Symptoms often start on the LEFT SIDE.
Symptoms always feel EXTREMELY SEVERE.
COPPERY TASTE – 'like old pennies.'

Mentals
Fear of strangers.
Easily tired.
Has to keep on the go.
Confused when ill.
Gets fixed ideas in mind.
Often uses the wrong words.
Maliciousness and spite.
Hate.

Modalities
Worse in the evenings and at night.
Worse in the cold.
Worse for vomiting.
BETTER FOR COLD DRINKS.
Better for perspiration.

Likes and dislikes
Likes cold drinks.
Likes warm food.

Physical features

Bluish tinge to mouth and lips.
Complains of slimy, metallic, coppery taste.
Constant need to lick lips, so that the tongue darts in and out, reptilean fashion.

Disease tendencies

All cramps – chest, abdomen, limbs or neuralgias.
Cramps often start in the fingers and toes.
Nausea, eased by drinking cold water.

Emotional tendencies

Fear of strangers.
Fixed ideas.
Hate.
Twitches and tics.

EQUISETUM

(Scouring-rush)

Not many mental symptoms.
EXCELLENT REMEDY FOR BED-WETTING IN CHILDREN.
Usually happens when have NIGHT-MARES or NIGHT TERRORS.

GELSEMIUM *****

(Yellow jasmine)

The classic 'flu' remedy.
There is great DROWSINESS with any ailment. There is nearly always the desire and need to lie down and sleep.
There is PROSTRATION, DIZZINESS and DULLNESS.
TIGHT, BURSTING HEADACHES.
Shivers up and down the spine.
Ailments from strong emotions – fear, anger, excitement.

Mentals

Wants to be left alone.

ANTICIPATORY ANXIETY – worries for days before an appointment, event, meeting.

Fear of death and of performing.

Excitable nature.

Confusion and drowsiness.

Unable to control muscles when ill.

Shakes and trembles with emotion.

Modalities

Worse for damp weather.

Worse before storms.

Worse for strong emotions.

WORSE FOR THINKING ABOUT AILMENTS.

Worse in mornings.

Better for bending backwards.

Better for being still.

Better for passing a lot of urine.

Likes and dislikes

LACK OF THIRST.

Physical features

Heavy eyelids.

Flushed appearance.

Dusky skin.

Disease tendencies

Paralytic conditions.

Migraine, especially producing occipital headaches.

Vertigo.

Respiratory infections and classical 'flu,' when there is great prostration.

Diarrhoea in anticipation of some dreaded appointment, event or meeting.

Emotional tendencies

Panic.

Anticipatory fear.

Bottled-up fear.
Fear of insects, spiders, death and of performing.
Ailments after anger.
Twitches and tics.

GRAPHITES *****
(Black lead)

Usually a female remedy.
Skin problems – tendency for wounds and cuts to FESTER.
CONSTIPATION with hard, knotty stools.
There is CHILLINESS.
ALTERNATING SKIN AND DIGESTIVE PROBLEMS.

Mentals
Timidity.
Indecisiveness.
Depression.
Tendency to fidget.
Anxiety.
MUSIC CAUSES WEEPINESS.
Often feels as if there are cobwebs on the face.
Guilt.

Modalities
Worse for heat.
Better in the dark.
Better for wrapping up.
Better for surrounding noise.
Better for eating.

Likes and dislikes
Dislikes meat.
Dislikes seafood and fish.
Dislikes sweets.
Dislikes hot drinks.

Physical features

Obesity.
Unhealthy skin.
Red faced.
Eyelids often red and swollen.
Sore nose with cracked skin around it.
Bad breath.

Disease tendencies

Styes.
Skin problems – all injuries tend to fester and take a long time to heal. Get cracked, dry skin around the nostrils, lips and behind the ears. May also get discharges which are thick, like honey. Crusting may take place afterwards.
Nail problems.
Stomach problems and indigestion, relieved by eating.
Nose-bleeds.
Chilblains.

Emotional tendencies

Lethargic or retarded depression.
Guilt.
Bulimia and ravenous appetite.
Premenstrual Syndrome.
Menopausal problems and post-menopausal depression.

HEPAR SULPH *****

(Calcium sulphide)

SENSITIVE TO ALL IMPRESSIONS – touch, pain and cold.
PERSPIRES EASILY, both day and night, although always likes to keep well covered.
Any skin problem seems to SUPPURATE, or gather pus.
CATARRHAL TENDENCY.
There is CHILLINESS.
SPLINTER-LIKE PAINS, especially of the throat.

Mentals

Irritable at the slightest provocation.
'Touchy,' even to the point of ferociousness.

Easily offended.
Speaks quickly.
When angry can easily go over the top.
Grumbling nature.
Can be quite resentful.
Violent potential.

Modalities
Worse for touch.
Worse for dry, cold winds.
Worse for draughts.
BETTER IN WET WEATHER.
BETTER FOR WRAPPING HEAD UP.
Better for eating.

Likes and dislikes
Likes pickles.
Likes vinegar.
Likes spices.
Dislikes fat.

Physical features
Cracked lower lip.
Perspires freely, but keeps wrapped up in spite of this.
Perspiration may have sour, offensive odour.
Skin discharges also tend to be offensive.

Disease tendencies
Skin problems which lead to infections.
Bedsores.
Ulcers of the skin.
Sore throats with swollen glands.
Eye infections.

Emotional tendencies
Irritability and anger.
Melancholia.
Violent potential.

Hyoscyamus
(Henbane)

ILL EFFECTS FROM UNSUCCESSFUL OR DISAPPOINTED LOVE.

Mentals
Suspiciousness of plots against him.
Talkative and may be obscene.
Tendency to want to uncover or expose the body.
Can feel very foolish.
May laugh at virtually anything.
Fear of animals.
Ritualistic behaviour, classically hand-washing.

Modalities
Worse at night.
Worse lying down.
Worse after food.
Better for bending.

Likes and dislikes
Nil in particular.

Physical features
Agitation, muscle tremors.

Disease tendencies
Coughs.
Convulsions.
Urine retention.

Emotional tendencies
Obsessive-compulsive behaviour, especially ritualistic hand-washing.
Fear of animals.
Suspicious.
Jealousy.
Guilt.
Ill effects of disappointed love.

HYPERICUM
(St John's Wort)

A great remedy for all puncturing or crushing injuries, eg, treading on nails, needles, splinters, trapped fingers and toes.
SPASMS after injury.
NEURALGIAS.

Mentals
Melancholic.
Depression after wounds, injuries or operations.
Dislike of heights.

Modalities
Worse for cold.
Worse for damp.
Worse for fog.
Worse for movement.
Worse for touch.
Better for bending the head back.
BETTER FOR RUBBING.

Likes and dislikes
Thirsty.
Likes wine.

Physical features
Nil in particular.

Disease tendencies
Wounds, punctures, crushes, concussions.
Coccydynia.
Haemorrhoids which are sensitive and bleed easily.
Neuralgia.

Emotional tendencies
Depression after crushing, wounds or operations.
Shock and acute nerve damage or injury.

IGNATIA
(St Ignatius Bean)

An excellent remedy for the ILL EFFECTS OF SHOCK, GRIEF OR FEAR.
Symptoms are often UNEXPECTED or CONTRADICTORY, eg, sore throats better for swallowing solids, indigestion better for eating, fevers better for keeping warm.
There is CHILLINESS.
There is great HYPERSENSITIVITY TO PAIN.
THROBBING, BURSTING and CRAMP-LIKE PAINS.

Mentals
Capricious – moods change rapidly and unexpectedly.
'Temperamentally mercurial.' Can flit from joy to depression and tearfulness extremely rapidly and almost without warning.
Hysterical depression.
Effects of GRIEF.
May sit and sigh a lot – even decades after the event.
Hypochondriasis.
Easily offended.
Jealousy.
Guilt.

Modalities
Worse in the mornings.
Worse in cold and open air.
Worse after food.
Worse for coffee.
BETTER WHILE EATING.
Better for changing position.
Better for lying on affected part.
Better for heat and the sun.

Likes and dislikes
Dislikes brandy.
Dislikes coffee.
Dislikes tobacco.
Likes sour food.
Likes vinegar and acidic food.

Physical features
May have involuntary twitching around the mouth.

Disease tendencies
Headaches, like a nail being driven into the skull.
Cramp-like pains.

Emotional tendencies
Fixed ideas.
Obsessive-compulsive behaviour.
Hypochondriasis.
Hysterical depression.
Hysterical problems. For example, difficulty swallowing, especially after a bereavement. This is the condition known as 'Globus Hystericus,' when it is harder to swallow liquids than solids.
'Psychosomatic problems.'
Grief reaction.
Irritability and hysterical anger outbursts.
Jealousy.
Guilt.
The ill effects of disappointed love.
Insomnia, despite frequent yawning.
Tobacco addiction.
Effects of acute shock.

IODUM
(Iodine)

Rapid metabolism.
Weight loss, despite good appetite. – THIS SYMPTOM MUST NOT BE IGNORED. A MEDICAL OPINION SHOULD BE SOUGHT TO ENSURE THAT A SERIOUS ILLNESS IS NOT IGNORED.

Mentals
Restless fear.
Anxiety and depression are often mixed.
May be a self-destructive tendency.
Suicidal thoughts may occur.
Has to keep busy.

Modalities
Worse when quiet.
Worse in the warm.
Better outdoors.

Likes and dislikes
Thirsty.
Ravenous hunger.

Physical features
Weight loss.
Flushes and blushes easily.
Gums may bleed easily.

Disease tendencies
Arthritis.
Respiratory infections.
Catarrhal deafness.

Emotional tendencies
Restless fear.
Agitated depression.
Self-destructive behaviour and suicidal thoughts.
Bulimia.

KALI PHOS *****
(Potassium phosphate)

THE NERVE SOOTHER.
Great PROSTRATION.
There is general WEAKNESS.
There is CHILLINESS.
There are yellow discharges.
PAIN IN LOWER NECK and BACK OF CHEST.

Mentals
Anticipatory anxiety.
Dread.
General lethargy.

Dislikes having to meet people, although hates being alone.
Easily sinks into depression.
Very nervous, TIMID and shy.
Irritability when forced out of shell, or backed into a corner.
Nightmares.
Despondency.
Poor memory and concentration when upset.
Fear of NERVOUS BREAKDOWN.

Modalities
Worse for worry.
Worse for physical exertion.
Worse for excitement.
Worse for eating.
Better for heat.
Better for movement.

Likes and dislikes
Likes ice-cold drinks.
Likes sweets.
Likes sour food.

Physical features
Thin, pale and always seems to look ill.
Blushes when stressed.
Tendency to perspire over the face and head.
Complains of pain in lower neck.

Disease tendencies
Tension headaches.
Dizziness from lying down.
Tinnitus.
Wet cough with yellow sputum.
Colds with yellow catarrh and nasal discharge.
Yellow diarrhoea coming on while eating.
Cystitis with yellow urine.

Emotional tendencies
Panic.
Anticipatory fear.

Lethargic or retarded depression.
Post Viral debility and depression.
Chronic Fatigue Syndrome.
Insomnia with night-mares or night terrors.

LACHESIS *****

(Bushmaster or Surukuku Snake Venom)

An excellent remedy for the menopause and after.
There is BLUENESS and PURPLISHNESS in all skin problems.
There is BLOATEDNESS – dislike of tight clothing or anything around the neck.
There is BURNING.
There is HYPERSENSITIVITY – to touch and noise.
TALKATIVE – tending to ramble on, constantly going off at tangents.
There is RESTLESSNESS.
Tendency towards LEFT-SIDED PROBLEMS, eg, sore throats start on the left.

Mentals

May feel full of sins.
Never at the best in the morning.
Never felt right since the menopause.
Fixed ideas about religion or philosophy.
Fear of burglars.
Suspicious of people and of the spouse.
Jealousy.
Nightmares.
There is post-menopausal depression.
Temper tantrums – can be quite vitriolic and deliberately hurtful.
Ailments come after grief.

Modalities

WORSE FOR SLEEP – always sleep into an aggravation of symptoms.
Worse for touch.
Worse for pressure.

Worse for motion.
Worse for heat.
Worse for hot drinks.
WORSE IN THE SPRING.
WORSE IN CLOUDY, OVERCAST WEATHER.
Better for warm applications.
Better after discharges, eg, of infection, or nose-bleeds.

Likes and dislikes

Likes coffee.
Likes alcohol.
Likes seafood.
Likes cold drinks.

Physical features

Blue or purplish face when ill.
Thin builds, maybe even seeming emaciated.
Pale face when well.

Disease tendencies

Sore throats – blue or purplish appearance. They start on the left side. The pain is usually out of proportion to the symptoms.
Asthma.
Hot flushes.
Headaches are typically hammering, worse for pressure and for sleep. May even wake up with a headache.
Palpitations, constricting anginal pains and a sensation of bloatedness.
Varicose veins – very blue and bloated.
Haemorrhoids – when they are large, blue or purple.

Emotional tendencies

Fear of burglars.
Fixed ideas.
Suspiciousness.
Hysterical depression.
Grief reaction.
Irritability and anger.
Jealousy.
Anger or jealousy after disappointed love.

Hate.
Premenstrual Syndrome.
Menopausal problems and post-menopausal depression.
Alcohol dependence.

LILIUM TIGRINUM
(Tiger-lily)

GYNAECOLOGICAL PROBLEMS.
There is HOTNESS with everything.

Mentals
Feels tormented.
Agitated depression.
Constant weepiness.
Feels the need at times to hit out or throw things. May also curse and swear.
May think obscene thoughts.
Has to keep busy, even if not achieving anything.
Increased sex drive before periods.

Modalities
WORSE FOR CONSOLATION.
Worse for warmth.
Better outdoors.

Likes and dislikes
Likes meat.
Thirsty.

Physical features
May be fair and with a tendency to be overweight.

Disease tendencies
Gynaecological problems.
Need to pass urine frequently.
Feeling as if the womb may fall out, especially when has period. May need to sit down and cross her legs.
Need to pass bowel motions frequently.

Emotional tendencies
Agitated depression.
Indifference.
Premenstrual Syndrome.

LYCOPODIUM *****

(Club Moss)

RIGHT-SIDED PROBLEMS.
Always looks older and more worried than years.
Symptoms worse between 4pm and 8pm.
Hair may go grey or fall out prematurely.
CUTTING AND BURNING PAINS.
There is CHILLINESS.

Mentals
Lack of self-confidence.
Anticipatory anxiety of events, yet when the time comes they usually cope very well.
Sexual fears.
Sensitive types.
Melancholia.
Agoraphobia.
Fears of being alone, darkness, death and ghosts.
Dislikes meeting strangers.
Forgetful of words when writing.
Irritable on waking.
Irritated by little things.
Dislikes contradiction.

Modalities
Worse for heat.
Worse for hot applications.
Worse for over-eating.
Better for motion.
Better for being uncovered.
Better for small meals.

Likes and dislikes
Likes sweet food.
Likes warm drinks.
Dislikes meat.
Dislikes cheese.
Dislikes seafood.

Physical features
Worried frown on forehead.
Intellectual types, eg, teachers, lawyers, doctors.
May go prematurely grey or bald.
Thin face, neck, chest, but well-nourished abdomen.
Tendency to stoop.
Often complains of one foot being hot while the other is cold.

Disease tendencies
Migraine.
Sore throats, starting on the right side, better for warm drinks.
Digestive problems, eg, flatulence, stomach ulcers, gall stones.
Kidney stones.
Hardening of the arteries.
Psoriasis.
Restless legs.
Dry vagina.

Emotional tendencies
Anticipatory fear.
Bottled-up fear.
Sexual fears, including erectile impotence and premature ejaculation.
Agoraphobia.
Fear of dark, death, crowds and performing.
Irritability.
Ailments after suppressed anger.
Jealousy.
Chronic Fatigue Syndrome.
Acute shock with fear of nervous breakdown.

MERCURIUS SOLUBILIS *****

(Black oxide of mercury)

There is WEAKNESS and WEARINESS of the limbs.
There is often a TREMOR and a tendency to STAMMER.
Infections are associated with glandular enlargement.
There is OFFENSIVENESS of all discharges.
There is ready PERSPIRATION which is offensive.
There is a metallic taste.
There is SENSITIVITY to TEMPERATURE CHANGES.
There are BURNING and CUTTING PAINS.

Mentals

General SLOWNESS of THOUGHT.
Poor memory.
Distrustful of others.
Fear of losing reason.
Fear of burglars.

Modalities

Worse for perspiring.
Worse for warmth of bed.
Worse at night.
Worse for damp.
Worse for lying on right side.

Likes and dislikes

Likes cold drinks.

Physical features

Offensive breath.
Flabby tongue showing the imprint of the teeth.
Poor mouth hygiene and spongy gums.
Skin moist from perspiration.
Face pale, dirty grey looking.

Disease tendencies

Sore throats with exudate and offensive breath.
Recurrent mouth problems.
Skin ulcers.
Bedsores.

Emotional tendencies
Fear of burglars.
Chronic Fatigue Syndrome and exhaustion.

Natrum Carbonicum

(Sodium carbonate)

EXHAUSTION AND DEBILITY IN THE HEAT.
WEAK ANKLES WHICH OFTEN 'TURN OVER.'

Mentals
Slow on the uptake.
Difficulty thinking and concentrating.
Melancholic.
Worrier.
Exhausted after mental exertion.
Over-critical of others.

Modalities
Worse for music.
Worse for the heat.
Worse for thunderstorms.
Worse for mental exertion.
Worse for draughts.
Worse for changes in the weather.
Better for moving.
Better for picking nose.

Likes and dislikes
Dislikes milk.

Physical features
Freckles, pale complexion, plump, with thick ankles.

Disease tendencies
Headaches from mental exertion.
Catarrh.
Dry cough.

Bowel problems with a desire to rush to the toilet.
Kidney problems.
Tendency to sprain ankles.

Emotional tendencies
Chronic Fatigue Syndrome.
Over-critical.
Nose-picking.

NATRUM MURIATICUM *****
(Salt)

There is CHILLINESS.
There may be a TREMOR.
Colds start with repeated sneezing.
There are SORE, CRAMPING and HAMMERING PAINS.

Mentals
Bottled up fear.
Agoraphobia.
Fear of burglars and thunderstorms.
Touchiness.
Hypochondriasis.
Agitated depression.
Ill effects or ailments from GRIEF.
Wants to weep but the tears won't come.
Broods on past slights.
Resentment.
Irritated by little things.
Dislikes sympathy.
Moody with changing emotions.
Guilt.
Hate.

Modalities
Worse in mornings.
Worse by the sea.
Worse for the sun.
Worse for thunderstorms.

Likes and dislikes
Craves salt.
Likes cold drinks.
Dislikes bread.

Physical features
Mapped tongue.
Cracked lower lip.
Oily skin and fine oily hair.
Thin neck and thin build, despite good appetite.

Disease tendencies
Cold sores.
Mouth ulcers.
Colds and respiratory infections.
Depression after grief or shock.
HAMMERING HEADACHES with preceding ZIG-ZAG VISION.
Palpitations.
Warts on hands and fingers.
Difficulty passing urine, especially if anyone is present.

Emotional tendencies
Bottled-up fear.
Agoraphobia.
Fear of burglars.
Fear of thunderstorms.
Hypochondriasis.
Agitated depression.
Grief reaction.
Irritability.
Outbursts of anger.
Guilt.
Depression or ailments after disappointed love.
Hate.
Anorexia.
Premenstrual Syndrome.
Acute shock.

NITRICUM ACIDUM *****
(Nitric acid)

General WEAKNESS, as with all 'acid' types.
There is CHILLINESS.
SPLINTER-LIKE PAINS.
Generalised SPIKINESS.

Mentals
Agitated depression.
Despair.
INDIFFERENCE.
Suspiciousness.
Obstinacy.
Irritability.
Vindictiveness.
Sensitivity to noise, pain and touch.
Fear of death.
Guilt.
Hate.

Modalities
Worse in the evenings and at night.
Worse for wind.
Worse for damp.
Worse for thunder.
Better for movement.

Likes and dislikes
Likes 'indigestible' food.
Likes salt.
Likes fat.

Physical features
Brown eyed.
May have been dark-haired.
Dark complexioned.
Cracks around the nose and mouth.

Disease tendencies
Tension headaches.
Mouth ulcers.
Sore throats which feel like splinters in the throat.
Respiratory infections with prickling sensation in the chest.
Offensive urine.
Constipation.
Anal fissures.
Haemorrhoids which have splinter-like pain persisting for long after the last motion was passed.
Warts which prickle, bleed and itch.

Emotional tendencies
Agitated depression.
Irritability.
Vindictiveness.
Guilt.
Hate.

NUX VOMICA *****
(Poison nut – contains strychnine)

Mainly a MALE REMEDY.
There is CHILLINESS.
There is HYPERSENSITIVITY – to noise, light and smell.
Ill effects of OVER-INDULGENCE – alcohol, rich food, coffee, tea, etc.
BURNING, CUTTING, ACHING and BURSTING PAINS.

Mentals
FASTIDIOUSNESS.
Quarrelsome.
Dislikes contradiction.
Dislikes being touched.
Always in a hurry.
Critical of others, always finding fault.
Fear of insects and spiders.
Fear of death.
Hypochondriasis.

Agitated depression.
Jealousy.
Guilt.

Modalities
Worse in the mornings.
Worse in windy weather.
Worse 2 hours after food.
Worse in open air.
Worse for the sun.
Better in the evening.
Better for sleep.
Better in damp, wet weather.
Better for pressure.

Likes and dislikes
Likes fat.
Likes rich food.

Physical features
Thin build.
Sedentary types who like 'good food, wine and company.'
Always in a hurry.
May be high-achievers.

Disease tendencies
Recurrent headaches and migraine.
Stomach problems – heartburn and indigestion.
Gastritis from over-indulgence.
Alcohol excess.
Hiccoughs.
Strangulated hernias.
Lumbago.
Constipation.

Emotional tendencies
Fear of death.
Fear of insects and spiders.
Hypochondriasis.
Agitated depression.

Irritability.
Short temper.
Jealousy.
Guilt.
Digestive problems starting after disappointed love.
Insomnia.
Premenstrual Syndrome.
Alcohol dependence.
Tobacco addiction.

Opium

(Dried seedbox of the poppy)

PAINLESSNESS.
EXTREMELY SLEEPY WITHOUT ANY RECOLLECTION OF DREAMS.
PERSPIRES EASILY.

Mentals

Desires nothing at all.
May be loss of consciousness.
Cannot understand the situation.
May be delirious.

Modalities

Worse for heat.
Worse during and after sleep.

Likes and dislikes

Loss of appetite.

Disease tendencies

Inactivity is the keynote. That is, inactivity of the bowel, the waterworks, the nervous system! Thus, constipation, retention of urine and paralysis.

Emotional tendencies

Panic, where one is rooted to the spot, or unable to think or move.
Acute shocks, both physical and mental.

PHOSPHORICUM ACIDUM
(Phosphoric acid)

There is general DEBILITY – mental first, followed by physical. Ill effects of grief, disappointment and having 'overdone it.'

Mentals
Mild nature.
Apathy.
Indifference.
Poor memory and confusion after disappointment.
Ill after suppressed anger or disappointed love.
Ill with grief or after grief.
Sexual fears after strong emotions.

Modalities
Worse for exertion.
Worse for loss of body fluids, eg, diarrhoea, perspiration, blood.
Worse for tight clothing.
Better for keeping warm.

Likes and dislikes
Likes juices.
Likes cold milk.
Dislikes sour things.

Physical features
May go grey or bald prematurely.
Blue rings around eyes.
Cracked lips.
Pale, earthy features.

Disease tendencies
Inflamed eyes.
Effects of grief.
General debility and weakness.
Nose-bleeds.
Back pain between the shoulder blades.
Flatulence or very pale diarrhoea.

Emotional tendencies
Grief reaction.
Indifference.
Ailments after suppressed anger.
Ill-effects of disappointed or unrequited love.
Sexual problems after strong emotions.
Chronic Fatigue Syndrome.
Acute shock.

PHOSPHORUS *****
(Phosphorus)

HYPERSENSITIVITY of all the senses.
Tendency to bleed easily, bright red blood.
BURNING PAINS.
Symptoms come and go suddenly.
Low resistance to coughs, colds, gastric infections.
Perspires easily on exertion, or in the mornings (especially on the lower lip).
There is CHILLINESS.
Emotions produce a TEMPERATURE.

Mentals
Artistic and creative.
Intelligent and imaginative.
Psychic or clairvoyant.
Easily angered, flares up.
Fearful of things which creep and crawl, thunderstorms, burglars, darkness and death.
Bottled-up fear.
Fixed ideas.
Agitated depression.
Indifference.
Apathy.
Great fatigue.
Likes sympathy.
Likes to be sympathetic to others.
Constantly needs reassurance.
Dislike of contradiction.
Hate.

Modalities

Better for eating – may have to eat in the night.
Generally better for warmth, but head symptoms better for cold.
Better for rubbing.

Likes and dislikes

Likes salt.
Likes spices.
Likes sour food.
Likes cold drinks which may be vomited as they warm up in the stomach.
Worse lying on the left.

Physical features

Tall and slim.
Brown eyes with long eyelashes.
Pale skin and dark hair, or red-haired and freckled.
Tendency to perspire on upper lip.

Disease tendencies

Glaucoma.
Styes.
Bleeding and bruising tendencies.
Vertigo.
Bursting headaches.
Recurrent respiratory infections.
Dry coughs.
Temperature and ailments after powerful emotions or excitement.

Emotional tendencies

Bottled-up fears.
Fear of burglars, darkness, death, ghosts and thunderstorms.
Fixed ideas about health.
Agitated depression.
Irritability.
Hate.
Insomnia and nightmares.
Thumb-sucking.
Twitches and tics.
Acute shock.

PICRIC ACIDUM
(Picric acid)

EXHAUSTION and MUSCULAR WEAKNESS.

Mentals
Lack of will-power.
Listless.

Modalities
Worse for exertion.
Feels weakness travelling upwards after exertion.

Likes and dislikes
Loss of appetite.

Physical features
Nil in particular.

Disease tendencies
Writer's palsy.
Anaemia.
Kidney problems.

Emotional tendencies
Chronic Fatigue Syndrome.
Anorexia and loss of appetite after viral infections.

PLATINA
(Platinum)

Mainly a female remedy.
NUMBNESS and COLDNESS.

Mentals
Arrogance.
Contempt for others.
Irritability.

Tremulousness.
Desire to hurt others – physically or mentally.

Modalities
Worse sitting.
Worse standing.
Worse in the evening.
Better for walking.

Likes and dislikes
Nil in particular.

Disease tendencies
Headaches after all sorts of prolonged emotions.
Abdominal colic.
Numbness with painful conditions.

Emotional tendencies
Arrogance.
Irritability.
Tremulousness.

PULSATILLA *****
(The wind flower)

Usually a FEMALE REMEDY.
There is CHILLINESS.
CHANGEABLE and CONTRADICTORY SYMPTOMS, eg, no two bouts of illness are the same; symptoms fluctuate hour by hour in a contradictory manner.
Perspiration on one side of the face.
NO THIRST.

Mentals
Mild and gentle.
Weeping tendency – for fear, misery or joy.

Laughs easily.
Tends to be quiet.
Bottled-up fear.
Claustrophobia.
Fear of darkness, death, ghosts and heights.
Fear of opposite sex.
Fixed ideas.
Obsessive-compulsive behaviour.
Likes sympathy.
Suspicious.
Irritable if slighted.
Religious nature. May feel full of sins.
Hysterical depression.
Jealousy.
Guilt.

Modalities
Worse for a stuffy atmosphere.
Worse for heat.
Better up and about, although when ill may feel better lying well-propped up in bed.
Better for a good weep.
Better for the open air.
Better for sympathy or consolation.
Better for motion.

Likes and dislikes
Dislikes fat.
Dislikes rich food.

Physical tendencies
'Girlish appearance' despite age.
Fair haired.
Blue eyed.
Tendency to put on weight.

Disease tendencies

Styes.
Catarrhal problems.
Varicose veins.
Incontinence.
Irritable bowel.
Skin problems.

Emotional tendencies

Bottled-up fear.
Claustrophobia.
Fear of darkness, death, ghosts, heights and opposite sex.
Fixed ideas.
Obsessive-compulsive behaviour.
Hysterical depression.
Grief reaction.
Jealousy.
Guilt.
Bulimia and binge-eating.
Premenstrual Syndrome.
Bed-wetting.
Thumb-sucking.
Acute shock.

RHODODENDRON

(Snow-rose)

An excellent rheumatic remedy.
ALWAYS WORSE BEFORE A STORM.
TEARING PAINS in neck and back.

Mentals

Dread of storms.
Fearful of thunder.
Poor memory generally.
Forgetful.
Agitated depression.

Modalities
Worse before storms.
All symptoms reappear in rough weather.
Better after storm breaks.
Better for warmth.
Better for eating.
Better immediately for moving.

Likes and dislikes
Nil in particular.

Physical features
Nil in particular.

Disease tendencies
Headaches, eye-aches, toothaches, stitch-like chest pains, all of which are worse before a storm.
Arthritis worse before a storm.
Neuralgic pains of the face and teeth.

Emotional tendencies
Fear of thunderstorms.
Agitated depression.

RHUS TOCICO DENDRON
(Poison ivy)

A great RHEUMATIC and SKIN remedy.
TEARING PAINS.
Mainly RIGHT-SIDED PROBLEMS
Ill effects of getting wet or chilled while perspiring.
Indeed, the ill effects of such an episode may have lingered for years.
There is RESTLESSNESS, so that the position has to be changed frequently.
Pains worse on starting to move, but get better as movement continues.
Stiffness on starting to move, but improving as movement continues.

Mentals
Melancholic.
Anxiety at night.
May contemplate suicide.
Fixation about being poisoned.
Hate.

Modalities
Worse during sleep.
Worse during cold, wet weather.
Worse after rain.
Worse at night.
Worse lying on back.
Worse lying on right side.
Better for warmth.
Better for walking.
Better for changing position.
Better for rubbing.
Better for stretching.

Likes and dislikes
Likes milk.
Always thirsty.

Physical features
Triangular red tip to the tongue.

Disease tendencies
Headaches after being in a draught or being chilled.
Inflamed eyes after being wet.
Joint pains better for movement.
Backache and lumbago.
Sprains and strains.
Sciatica.
Blistering skin problems.
Cold sores.
Shingles.

Emotional tendencies
Fixations, particularly about being poisoned.
Hate.

SABADILLA
(Cevadilla seed)

CHILLINESS.

Mentals
Timid.
Bizarre body image.
Convinced that he is ill.

Modalities
Worse for cold drinks.
Worse for the full moon.
Better for warm food.

Likes and dislikes
Likes sweets.
Likes hot food and drink.

Physical features
Red eyelids.
Dry skin.
Tremulous.

Disease tendencies
Recurrent colds.
Stomach cramps.
Hay fever and rhinitis.
Left-sided sore throat.

Emotional tendencies
Altered body image.
Bulimia.

SEPIA *****
(Cuttlefish ink)

Usually a FEMALE REMEDY.
DRAGGING DOWN SENSATION, as if the womb is about to

prolapse. Often wants to cross the legs to get rid of the sensation.

May be very depressed and withdrawn, but COMES ALIVE WITH EXERTION, classically dancing.

There is CHILLINESS, although flushes are common.

BURNING OR THROBBING PAINS.

Mentals

SLOWNESS.

INDIFFERENCE to loved ones.

Lethargic depression.

Tiredness and weakness.

Aggression to loved ones.

Irritable and easily offended.

Weepiness.

Feels that cannot cope.

Wants to get away from it all.

Likes a good cry.

Dislikes sympathy and consolation.

Dislikes company, but hates being alone. Tends to avoid crowds.

Resentful of people who interfere or fuss after them.

Fear of disease and fixed ideas about disease.

Modalities

Worse for tobacco.

Worse before a storm.

Worse for too much sedentary work.

Better for food.

Better for exertion, especially dancing.

Better for sleep.

Likes and dislikes

Dislikes meat.

Dislikes milk.

Dislikes fat.

Likes vinegar.

Likes spices.

Physical features

Thin build.
Yellowish 'saddle' across the bridge of the nose, or a 'butterfly' rosy colouration across the cheeks and nose. Cracked lower lip.
May be a brunette.

Disease tendencies

Migraine and headaches, better for sleep.
Menopausal problems.
Constipation, with a ball-like sensation in the back passage.
Haemorrhoids.

Emotional tendencies

Fixation about disease.
Indifference.
Lethargic or retarded depression.
Grief reaction.
Irritability.
Depression or indifference after disappointed love.
Chronic Fatigue Syndrome.
Premenstrual Syndrome.
Menopausal problems and post-menopasal depression.

SILICEA *****

(Flint)

SLOW HEALING.
There is CHILLINESS.
There is offensive perspiration of the head and feet.
Prone to colds and respiratory infections.
BURNING, CUTTING, SORE AND THROBBING PAINS.

Mentals

Dread of failure.
Lack of self-confidence.
Timidity.
Anticipatory anxiety of events and appointments.

Exhausted after conversation.
Dislikes talking.
Fixed ideas about pins – wants to find them and count them. Basically fears them.

Modalities

Worse for draughts.
Better for warmth.
Better for wrapping up.

Likes and dislikes

Likes cold food.
Always thirsty.
Dislikes meat.
Dislikes milk.

Physical features

Thin, delicate 'China-doll' appearance (prominent foreheads).
Small sweaty hands and feet.
White spots on the nails.

Disease tendencies

Boils and septic tendencies.
Bone pains and bone problems.
Headaches, better for wrapping up.
Chest infections that are slow to clear.
History of TB.
Constipation – when the motion can only be partially expelled and tends to slip back.

Emotional tendencies

Fear of performing.
Anticipatory fear.
Fixations about small objects and counting.

SPIGELIA

(Pinkroot)

A remedy of DEBILITY in anaemia and rheumatism.
There is CHILLINESS.
There is sensitivity to touch.

Mentals
Fear of sharp objects.

Modalities
Worse for touch.
Worse for motion.
Worse for noise.
Worse for washing.
Better for lying on the right side with the head propped high.
Better for breathing in.

Likes and dislikes
Nil in particular.

Physical features
Pale, debilitated looking.

Disease tendencies
Glaucoma.
Facial neuralgias.
Palpitations and angina, and angina with palpitations.
Both of these heart symptoms seem to be relieved by drinking hot water.

Emotional tendencies
Insomnia with violent palpitations. They may be so severe that a sleeping partner is awoken.

STAPHISAGRIA *****
(Stavesacre)

AILMENTS FROM SUPPRESSED ANGER OR INDIGNATION.
HYPERSENSITIVE TO TOUCH.
Good remedy after any cuts, eg, operations.

Mentals

Violent flare-ups of temper which tries to suppress.
Aggressiveness.
Hypochondraical – always thinking about their illness and their symptoms.
Very sensitive.
Easily offended.
Likes solitude.
Resentment.
Jealousy.
Pride.

Modalities

Worse for the cold.
Worse for touch.

Likes and dislikes

Likes tobacco.
Likes milk.

Physical features

Sunken eyes, itchy, flaky eyelids. May have eczema with thickish crusts.

Disease tendencies

Good post-operative remedy to hasten healing after the body has been cut or incised.
Headaches from anger or strong emotions.
Styes.
Colic after anger.
Prostate enlargement.
Eczema.
Warts around the back passage.
Skin problems which start after anger.

Emotional tendencies

Over-sensitiveness.
Irritability and anger.
Dislike of criticism.
Violent temper which they try to suppress.

Jealousy.
Pride.
Disappointed love may lead to anger, violent outbursts or illness (if suppressed).

STRAMONIUM
(Thorn-apple)

PAINLESSNESS.
EXPRESSIONLESSNESS.

Mentals
Talkative.
Tendency to sing, swear and laugh.
Rapid mood changes.
May be violent and aggressive.
Dislikes solitude.
Hates the darkness and has to have a light on.
Dislikes the sight of water or glimmering surfaces.

Modalities
Worse for the darkness.
Worse for own company.
Worse for looking at bright, or shimmering, or glimmering objects.
Better for company.
Better for light rooms.

Likes and dislikes
All food seems 'tasteless! – like straw!'

Disease tendencies
All delirious conditions.

Emotional tendencies
Fear of animals.
Fear of the dark.
Moodswings.
Jealousy.
Violent anger.

SULPHUR *****
(Sulphur)

BURNING OR ITCHING.
REDNESS of affected parts.
OFFENSIVENESS OF ODOURS.
DIRTINESS – there will always be at least one aspect of the appearance which has been left. For example, if a nice new suit is worn the shoes may be left unpolished. Neatness and cleanliness is not high on their order of priorities. There is PERIODICITY, in that symptoms seem to come on every seven days during an illness.
Skin complaints alternate with internal problems.
There is FIDGETING – they are unable to stand, sit or lie still. They have to lean, change feet, etc.
There is general HOTNESS.

Mentals
Philosophical nature.
Selfish and self-centred.
Argumentative and aggressive.
Sensitive to odours, although they themselves may have offensive perspiration which they are oblivious to.
Dislike getting washed or bathed, although may be fond of swimming.
Claustrophobia.
Fear of ghosts and heights.
Fixed ideas about the body.
Lethargic depression.
Hate of oppressive regimes, injustice, etc.

Modalities
Worse for washing or bathing.
Worse for the heat of the bed.
Worse at 11am, when gets a sinking feeling in the stomach.
Worse for standing or sitting still.
Better for the open air.

Likes and dislikes
Always thirsty.
Always hungry.
Likes fat.
Likes sweets.
Likes coffee and other stimulants.
Likes alcohol.

Physical features
Red lipped.
Dirty appearance.
Lean, lanky, 'ragged philosopher' appearance.
Sometimes may be more like a well-rounded bon viveur.
Always leaves at least one article of clothing, or one aspect of appearance unkempt.

Disease tendencies
Glaucoma.
Catarrhal problems.
Skin problems of all sorts.
BURNING PAINS.
Burning feet.
Early morning diarrhoea which makes them get out of bed.
Constipation.
Haemorrhoids – red, burning and itching.
Lumbago on getting up in the morning or when turning.
Alcoholism.
Gout.

Emotional tendencies
Claustrophobia.
Fear of ghosts and heights.
Fixed ideas about the body.
Lethargic or retarded depression.
Hate of oppression and injustice.
Insomnia.
Bulimia.
Menopausal problems and post-menopausal depression.
Alcohol dependence.
Nose-picking.

Thumb-sucking.
Tobacco addiction.

TARENTULA HISPANIA
(Spanish spider)

CONSTRICTING SENSATIONS.

Mentals
Restlessness.
Sudden mood swings.
Fixed ideas and destructive impulses.
Sensitive to music.
High sex drive.

Modalities
Worse for motion.
Worse for noise.
Worse for seeing others in trouble.
Better for the open air.

Likes and dislikes
Nil in particular.

Physical features
Nil in particular.

Disease tendencies
Vertigo.
Weakness of the legs.
Constricting pains.

Emotional tendencies
Fixed ideas with destructive behaviour.

Thuja Occidentalis
(Arbor vitae)

A great WART REMEDY.
There is CHILLINESS.
There is a sweet odour to the perspiration which is often profuse over uncovered parts.

Mentals
Anxiety.
Weeps easily.
Makes mistakes in reading and writing.
Can get odd ideas fixed in their minds, eg, as if the body is rigid, brittle like glass. As if something is living inside them.
Fear of strangers.

Modalities
Worse for the heat of the bed.
Worse at night.
Worse for cold.

Likes and dislikes
Dislikes potatoes.
Dislikes meat.
Dislikes fat.
LOVES TEA.

Physical features
Tendency to warts and warty growths.

Disease tendencies
Headaches, as if a nail is being driven into skull.
Styes.
Nasal polyps.
Haemorrhoids.
Nail problems.
Warts and warty growths anywhere.

Emotional tendencies
Fear of strangers.
Strange fixed ideas.
Loss of appetite.
Anorexia with strange ideas about body image.
Twitches and tics.

VALERIAN

(Valerian)

HYSTERICAL SPASMS.

Mentals
Changeableness.
Claustrophobia.
Hysterical outbursts.
Hysterical depression.
Hypochondriasis.
Over-sensitivity.

Modalities
Worse for sleep.
Worse for cold draughts.

Likes and dislikes
Likes to eat when nauseated.

Physical features
Nil in particular.

Disease tendencies
Hysterical spasms.
Earache from exposure to draughts.
Abdominal cramps.
Jerking legs.

Emotional tendencies
Claustrophobia
Hysterical depression.

Irritability.
Hypochondriasis.

Veratrum Album
(White Hellebore)

COLDNESS.
BLUENESS.
There may be collapse.
COLD PERSPIRATION ON BROW.

Mentals
Melancholy and lethargic depression.
May be drowsiness.
Sulky and indifferent.
Acute upsets when has the impulse and desire to tear or cut things up.
Guilt feelings.

Modalities
Worse for wet weather.
Worse at night.
Better for walking.
Better for warmth.

Likes and dislikes
Likes cold water.
Craving for fruit.
Likes salt.

Physical features
Sunken eyes and pointed nose.

Disease tendencies
Profuse vomiting.
Constipation.
Chronic bronchitis.
Palpitations.

Emotional tendencies
Fixations about tearing and cutting things up.
Lethargic depression.
Guilt.

ZINCUM METALLICUM
(Zinc)

SENSITIVE TO NOISES AND TALKING.
RESTLESS LEGS.
There is CHILLINESS.
CRAMPING PAINS
Lack of vitality.
Twitching tendency.
Anaemia is common.

Mentals
Depression.
Poor memory.
Feels as if the head will fall to one side, because it is so heavy.
Exhaustion.

Modalities
Worse after dinner.
Worse for wine.
Better while eating.
Better after discharges, from nose, wounds etc.

Likes and dislikes
Always hungry in late morning, with a ravenous appetite.

Disease tendencies
Chilblains.
Cramps of all sorts.
Varicose veins.
Restless legs.

Emotional tendencies
Chronic Fatigue Syndrome.
Bulimia.
Alcohol dependence.
Twitches and tics.

Therapeutic Index

An A–Z of common emotional symptoms and conditions, with the remedies most likely to help.

AGGRESIVENESS – Bell, Hep sulph, Nux vom, Staph, Sulph.
AGORAPHOBIA – Acon, Arn, Ars alb, Lyc, Nat mur. (See also FEAR)
ALCOHOL DEPENDENCE – Acon, Ars alb, Lach, Nux vom, Sulph, Zinc.
ALCOHOL, ILL EFFECTS – Ars alb, Bar carb, Nux vom, Sulph.
ALUMINIUM, ILL EFFECTS – Alum, Lyc.
ANGER – Acon, Bell, Cham, Hep sulph, Ign, Nux vom, Sep, Staph, Sulph.
ANGER, ILL EFFECTS – Apis, Bry, Cham, Coloc, Gel, Ign, Lyc, Nux vom, Phos Ac, Staph, Stram.
ANOREXIA – Alum, Aur, Caust, Nat mur, Pic Ac, Thuj.
APATHY – Apis, Chin, Nat mur, Phos, Puls, Sep.
APPETITE, POOR – See ANOREXIA.
APPETITE, INCREASED, RAVENOUS – See BULIMIA.
APPREHENSION – Arg nit, Ars alb, Gels, Lyc, Sil. (See also FEAR)
ANTICIPATORY ANXIETY – Arg nit, Gels, Kali phos, Lyc. (See also FEAR)
ANXIETY – See under APPREHENSION and FEARS.
ARROGANCE – Lyc, Plat, Sulph, Verat.

BED-WETTING – Arg nit, Bell, Equis, Puls.
BEREAVEMENT – See GRIEF.
BODY IMAGE DISORDERS – See ANOREXIA and BULIMIA.
BOTTLED-UP FEAR – Caust, Gels, Lyc, Nat mur, Phos, Puls. (See also FEAR)
BULIMIA – Ammon carb, Arg nit, Calc carb, Chin, Graph, Iod, Phos, Puls, Sabad, Sulph, Zinc.

CHANGEABLE – Ign, Lyc, Nux vom, Puls.
CHRONIC FATIGUE SYNDROME – Alum, Ammon carb, Anac, Calc carb, Chin, Kali phos, Lyc, Merc sol, Nat carb, Phos ac, Pic ac, Sep, Zinc. (See also EXHAUSTION)
CLAUSTROPHOBIA – Arg nit, Carbo veg, Puls, Sulph, Valer. (See also FEAR)
COMPULSIONS – See FIXATIONS AND IMPULSES.
CONSOLATION, WORSE FOR – Ign, Nat mur, Sep. BETTER FOR – Puls.
CURSING – Anac, Hyos.

DEBILITY – If sustained a medical opinion should be sought. See CHRONIC FATIGUE SYNDROME and EXHAUSTION.
DESPAIR – Acon, Ars alb, Bry, Calc carb, Nux vom, Sep.
DEPRESSION, AGITATED – Ars alb, Aur, Bell, Iod, Lil tig, Nat mur, Nit ac, Nux vom, Phos, Rhus tox.
DEPRESSION, HYSTERICAL – Cimic, Ign, Lach, Puls, Valer.
DEPRESSION, LETHARGIC or RETARDED – Calc carb, Chin, Graph, Kali phos, Sep, Sulph, Verat.
DREAMS, FEARFUL – Acon, Alum, Ars alb, Bar carb, Calc carb, Nat mur, Phos, Puls, Thuj.
  OF BEING CHASED – Sil, Sulph.
  OF THE DEAD – Ars alb, Thuj.
  OF FLYING – Apis.
  OF MURDER – Arn, Nat mur.

EATING DISORDERS – See ANOREXIA and BULIMIA and BODY IMAGE DISORDERS

EXCITEMENT – ILLNESS AFTER – Acon, Arg nit, Aur, Coff, Graph, Nat mur, Phos ac.
EXHAUSTION, MENTAL – Anac, Calc carb, Kali phos, Nat carb, Phos ac, Pic ac, Sep, Zinc.

FEAR, ANTICIPATORY – Arg nit, Gels, Kali phos, Lyc.
BOTTLED-UP – Caust, Gels, Lyc, Nat mur, Phos, Puls.
RESTLESS – Ars alb, Bry, Calc carb, Iod, Lyc, Nat mur.
(See also PHOBIAS)
FIXATIONS – Acon, Anac, Arg nit, Ars alb, Aur, Cup met, Hyos, Ign, Lach, Phos, Puls, Rhus tox, Sep, Sil, Sulph, Tarent, Thuj, Verat. (See also impulses)

GRIEF – Ars alb, Aur, Caust, Ign, Lach, Nat mur, Phos ac, Puls, Sep.
GUILT – Anac, Ars alb, Aur, Bell, Caust, Cocc, Coff, Graph, Hyos, Ign, Nat mur, Nit ac, Nux vom, Puls, Verat.

HATE – Anac, Aurum, Calc carb, Cup Met, Lach, Nat mur, Nit ac, Phos, Rhus tox, Sulph,
HOME-SICKNESS – Cap.
HUNGER, RAVENOUS – See BULIMIA.
HYPOCHONDRIASIS – Ars alb, Aur, Calc carb, Ign, Nat mur, Nux vom, Val.
HYSTERIA – Aur, Caust, Gels, Ign, Lach, Nat mur, Puls, Sep.

IMPULSES (Including compulsions to check, wash-hands repeatedly, ritualistic behaviour, etc.)
– Arg nit, Ars alb, Hyos, Puls, Sil, Sulph, Tarent, Verat.
IMPOTENCE – See SEXUAL FEARS
INDIFFERENCE – Apis, Chin, Nat mur, Phos, Puls, Sep.
INJURIES, SHOCK – See SHOCK and TRAUMA.
INSOMNIA – Arn, Ars alb, Bell, Chin, Coff, Ign, Nux vom, Phos, Spig, Sulph.
IRRITABILITY – Anac, Ars alb, Aur, Bell, Bry, Cap, Cham, Chin, Coloc, Hep sulph, Ign, Lach, Lyc, Nat mur, Nit ac, Nux vom, Phos, Plat, Puls, Sep, Staph. Thuj.

JEALOUSY – Apis, Ars alb, Calc carb, Hyos, Ign, Lach, Lyc, Nux vom, Puls, Staph, Stram.

LOVE, EFFECTS OF DISAPPOINTED OR UNREQUITED – Aur, Calc phos, Caust, Cimic, Coff, Hyos, Ign, Lach, Nat mur, Nux vom, Phos ac, Sep, Staph.

MEMORY PROBLEMS – Alum, Anac, Apis, Bar carb, Cocc, Lyc, Rhod.
MENOPAUSE PROBLEMS – Aur, Graph, Lach, Sep, Sulph.
MENTAL EXHAUSTION – See EXHAUSTION, MENTAL and CHRONIC FATIGUE SYNDROME.

NAIL-BITING – Ammon br, Arg nit, Arum tri.
NIGHT-MARES and NIGHT TERRORS – Acon, Equis, Kali phos, Lach, Sulph, Valer, Zinc. (See also INSOMNIA)
NOISE, SENSITIVE TO – Acon, Bell, Chin, Coff, Nux vom, Sep.
NOSE-PICKING – Arum tri, Cina, Nat carb, Sulph.

OFFENDED EASILY – Alum, Apis, Ars alb, Aur, Calc carb, Caust, Chin, Graph, Lyc, Nux vom, Puls, Sep, Spig.
OVER-SENSITIVE – See OFFENDED EASILY

PALPITATIONS – Ars alb, Bar carb, Nat mur, Rhus tox, Spig.
PANIC – Acon, Gels, Kali phos, Op.
PHOBIA, OF ANIMALS – Caust, Chin, Hyos, Stram.
OF BURGLARS – Ars alb, Lach, Merc sol, Nat mur, Phos.
OF CROWDS – See AGORAPHOBIA.
OF DARK – Acon, Calc carb, Caust, Lyc, Phos, Puls, Stram.
OF DEATH – Acon, Apis, Arg nit, Ars alb, Bry, Calc carb, Caust, Gels, Lyc, Nux vom, Phos, Puls.
OF ENCLOSED SPACES – See CLAUSTROPHOBIA.
OF GHOSTS – Acon, Ars alb, Caust, Lyc, Phos, Puls, Sulph.
OF HEIGHTS – Arg nit, Puls, Sulph.
OF INSECTS AND SPIDERS – Arg nit, Gels, Nux vom.
OF PERFORMING IN PUBLIC – Arg nit, Caust, Gels, Lyc, Sil.
OF STRANGERS – Bar carb, Carb veg, Caust, Cup met, Thuj.
OF THUNDERSTORMS – Nat mur, Phos, Rhod.

POST-MENOPAUSAL DEPRESSION – See MENOPAUSAL PROBLEMS
PREMENSTRUAL SYNDROME – Calc carb, Caust, Graph, Lach, Lil tig, Nat mur, Nux vom, Puls, Sep.
PRIDE, FULL OF – Caust, Cup met, Lach, Lyc, Plat, Staph, Stram, Sulph, Thuj, Verat.
PRIDE, WOUNDED – Arg nit, Aur, Coloc, Graph, Lyc, Nux vom, Puls, Sep, Spig, Staph, Sulph, Verat.

RESTLESSNESS – Acon, Anac, Arg nit, Bell, Bry, Calc carb, Calc phos, Cimic, Coloc, Cup met, Hyos, Kali phos, Lil tig, Lyc, Merc sol, Nux vom, Puls, Rhus tox, Sil, Sep, Staph, Stram, Sulph, Tarent, Zinc.
RUDENESS – Anac, Hyos, Lyc, Nux vom, Sram, Verat.

SADNESS – See DEPRESSION
SEXUAL FEARS – FEMALE – VAGINISMUS – Bell, Cact.
– MALE – IMPOTENCE – Arg nit, Lyc, Phos ac.
SHOCK – Acon, Ign, Lyc, Nat mur, Op, Phos ac, Phos, Puls.
SLEEP PROBLEMS – See INSOMNIA
SUICIDAL THOUGHTS – WHENEVER THESE OCCUR A MEDICAL OPINION SHOULD BE SOUGHT. Ars alb, Aur, Calc carb, Chin, Cimic, Hep sulph, Lach, Merc sol, Puls, Sep, Stram.
SUSPICIOUSNESS – Acon, Ars alb, Bar carb, Caust, Lach, Lyc, Puls, Rhus tox, Stram, Sulph.

TALKATIVENESS – Hyos, Lach, Stram.
TEARFULNESS – Apis, Ign, Nat mur, Puls, Rhus tox, Sep.
TEETH-GRINDING – Apis, Ars, Bell, Cina, Hyos, Stram, Verat, Zinc.
THREATENING BEHAVIOUR – Hep sulph, Stram, Tarent.
THUMB-SUCKING – Ars alb, Phos, Puls, Sulph.
TICS and TWITCHES – Acon, Arg nit, Cup met, Gels, Phos, Thuj, Zinc.
TIMIDITY – Calc carb, Gels, Lyc, Phos, Sep.
TOBACCO DEPENDENCE – Ars alb, Ign, Nux vom, Sulph.
TRAUMA, SHOCK – Acon, Arn, Carb veg, Hyper, Op.
TREMORS – Since this may herald the onset of a cerebro-

vascular disease or a neurological condition like Parkinson's Disease, a medical opinion should be sought.

WEEPINESS - See TEARFULNESS

Useful Addresses

The following organisations will be able to supply lists of registered homoeopathic practitioners.

The British Homoeopathic Association,
27a Devonshire Street,
London EC1N 1RJ

The Faculty of Homoeopathy,
The Royal London Homoeopathic Hospital,
Great Ormond Street,
London WC1N 3HR

The Hahnemann Society,
The Humane Education Centre,
2 Powys Place,
Great Ormond Street,
London WC1N 3HT

The Society of Homoeopaths,
2 Artizan Road,
Northampton NN1 4HU

The United Kingdom Homoeopathic Medical Association,
6 Livingstone Road,
Gravesend,
Kent DA12 5DZ

Homoeopathic Pharmacies

Many chemists and health shops now carry a range of the Bach Flower Remedies and the commonest homoeopathic remedies. The following pharmacies and manufacturers will usually supply products through the post.

Ainsworths,
38 New Cavendish Street,
London W1M 7LH

Freemans,
7 Eaglesham Road,
Clarkston,
Glasgow G76 7BU

Galen Pharmacy,
Lewell Mill,
West Stafford,
Dorchester,
Dorset DT2 8AN

A Nelson & Co Ltd,
73 Duke Street,
Grosvenor,
London W1M 6BY

Weleda (UK) Ltd, (Manufacturer)
Heanor Road,
Ilkeston,
Derbyshire DE7 8DR

Homoeopathic Hospitals

The Bristol Homoeopathic Hospital,
Cotham Road,
Cotham,
Bristol BS6 6JU

Glasgow Homoeopathic Hospital,
1000 Great Western Road,
Glasgow G12 0RN

The Department of Homoeopathic Medicine,
The Liverpool Clinic,
Mossley Hill Hospital,
Park Avenue,
Liverpool L18 8BU

The Royal London Homoeopathic Hospital,
Great Ormond Street,
London WC1

Tunbridge Wells Homoeopathic Hospital,
Church Road,
Tunbridge Wells,
Kent TN1 1JU

ABROAD

AFRICA

African Homoeopathic Medical Federation,
PO Box 131,
Nempi,
Oru L.G.A.,
Imo State,
Nigeria,
Africa

INDIA

Hahnemannian Society of India,
476 Gautam Nagar,
New Delhi 110 949
India

New Zealand

New Zealand Homoeopathic Society,
PO 2939,
Auckland,
New Zealand

South Africa

Homoeopathic Society of South Africa,
PO Box 9658,
Johannesburg 2000,
South Africa

Australia

Australian Institute of Homoeopathy,
21 Bulah Close,
Berowra Heights,
Sydney NSW 2082

Brauer Biotherapies (Pharmacy)
1 Para Road,
Tanunda,
South Australia, 5352

France

Liga Medicorm Homoeopathica Internationalis,
1068 21025 Dijon Cedex,
France

Dolisos, (Manufacturer)
62, Rue Beaubourg 75003,
Paris,
France

USA

American Foundation for Homeopathy,
1508 S Garfield,
Alhambra,
CA 91801,
USA

Homeopathic Educational Services,
2124 Kittredge Street,
Berkeley,
CA 94704,
USA

National Center for Homeopathy,
801 N. Fairfax, Suite 306,
Alexandria,
Virginia, 22314,
USA

Santa Monica Drug Co, (Pharmacy)
1513 Fourth Street,
Santa Monica,
CA 90401,
USA

Standard Homeopathic Company, (Pharmacy)
210 West 131st Street,
Los Angeles,
CA 90061,
USA

USEFUL ORGANIZATIONS

The following organizations may be able to supply helpful information about their specific areas of concern.

Action on Smoking and Health (ASH),
27 Mortimer Street,
London W1N 7RH

Alcoholics Anonymous,
PO Box 514,
11 Redcliffe Gardens,
London SW10 9BQ

Anorexic Aid,
The Priory Centre,
11 Priory Road,
High Wycombe,
Bucks HP13 6SL

National Association for Premenstrual Syndrome,
25 Market Street,
Guildford,
Surrey GU1 4LB

Phobics Society,
4 Cheltenham Road,
Chorlton-cum-Hardy,
Manchester M21 1QN

TRANX (Tranquilliser Recovery and New Existence),
17 Peel Road,
Harrow,
Middlesex HA3 7QX

Index

Physical symptoms, feelings and emotions all play their part in homoeopathic diagnosis and the entries in this index use the words shown in the text cross referenced to similar and related terms. Subheadings have been used to break up long lists of page numbers wherever possible. For reasons of space mentals, modalities, physical features and disease tendencies from the Materia Medica have only been indexed when they are characteristic features (see p. 174), but all likes/dislikes and modalities are included. Major entries are shown in bold.

T